Innovation in Osteogenesis Research

Edited by Ziyad S. Haidar

Published in London, United Kingdom

Innovation in Osteogenesis Research
http : //dx . doi . org/10 . 5772/intechopen . 1001703
Edited by Ziyad S . Haidar

Contributors
Ayesha Bashir , Betsy Joseph , Nandita Suresh , Naveeda Bashir , Qurrat ul Ain , Rana Muhammad Zeeshan , Sukumaran Anil , Tuomas Waltimo , Wajahat Sohail , Ziyad S . Haidar

First published in London , United Kingdom , 2025 by IntechOpen
IntechOpen is the global imprint of INTECHOPEN LIMITED , registered in England and Wales , registration number : 11086078 , 167-169 Great Portland Street , London , W1W 5PF , United Kingdom

For EU product safety concerns : IN TECH d . o . o . , Prolaz Marije Krucifikse Kozulić 3 , 51000 Rijeka , Croatia , info@intechopen . com or visit our website at intechopen . com .

British Library Cataloguing-in-Publication Data
A catalogue record for this book is available from the British Library

Innovation in Osteogenesis Research
Edited by Ziyad S . Haidar
p . cm .
Print ISBN 978-1-83769-646-8
Online ISBN 978-1-83769-645-1
eBook (PDF) ISBN 978-1-83769-647-5

If disposing of this product , please recycle the paper responsibly .

Meet the editor

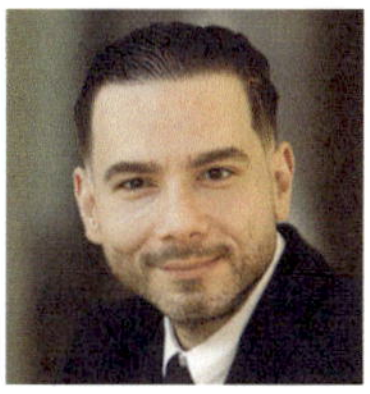

Ziyad S. Haidar is a Full Professor of NanoBioEngineering and the Faculty of Dentistry Scientific Director at Universidad de los Andes (UANDES) in Santiago, Chile. Prof. Dr. Haidar is the Founder and CEO of the BioMAT'X I+D+I/HAiDAR R&D&I LABs Chile), Head of BioHealth Innovation at Centro de Investigación e Innovación Biomédica (CiiB) and a Faculty member in the Masters and Doctoral Programs (BioMedicine) at the Faculty of Dentistry, and Faculty of Medicine at UANDES. Haidar is also a visiting professor at institutions such as Universidad de La Frontera (UFRO- Temuco) and the University of Montreal. Haidar is an oral and cranio-maxilla-facial surgeon with a Ph.D. in nanobiomaterials and bio-engineering from McGill University, an MBA from Concordia University, and completed post-doctoral training at the Montréal Shriners Hospital, MUHC, Montréal, QC, Canada.

Contents

Preface **IX**

Chapter 1 **1**
Introductory Chapter: Forming and Regenerating Bone – The Science of Osteogenesis, R&D&I
by Ziyad S. Haidar

Chapter 2 **11**
NSAIDs Effect on Bone Healing
by Rana Muhammad Zeeshan

Chapter 3 **35**
Bone Development and Growth
by Ayesha Bashir, Qurrat ul Ain, Naveeda Bashir and Wajahat Sohail

Chapter 4 **63**
Hereditary Hemorrhagic Telangiectasia (HHT)/Osler-Weber-Rendu Syndrome: A Review on Contemporary Knowledge, Its Accompanying Clinical Manifestations, Diagnostics, and Oro-Dental Management Plan
by Ziyad S. Haidar

Chapter 5 **87**
Elevated Non-fasting Plasma Total Homocysteine Level is Associated with Alveolar Bone and Tooth Loss: Insights for Osteogenic Innovations
by Ziyad S. Haidar

Chapter 6 **101**
Phyto-Nanoparticles in Osteogenesis
by Nandita Suresh, Betsy Joseph, Tuomas Waltimo and Sukumaran Anil

Preface

Bone, an extraordinary and dynamic organ, is fundamental to the human body's structure, function, and overall health. It provides structural support, protects vital organs, facilitates mobility, and regulates mineral homeostasis. Beyond its mechanical roles, bone is a living connective tissue capable of remarkable self-repair and remodeling, driven by a delicate balance between the activities of osteoblasts, osteoclasts, and osteocytes. Biochemical signals, mechanical forces, and systemic factors such as hormones, nutrition, and environmental influences regulate this equilibrium. Bone development and growth are tightly controlled processes that begin in the embryonic stage and continue through adulthood. The intricate orchestration of genetic, molecular, and cellular interactions ensures the formation of a robust skeletal framework while allowing for its dynamic adaptation to mechanical demands throughout life. However, disruptions to these processes can lead to congenital anomalies, growth disorders, or an impaired ability to regenerate and repair. Osteogenesis, the process of bone formation, is central not only to skeletal development but also to bone repair, regeneration, and restoration. While bone possesses an inherent capacity to heal itself, this ability is often compromised in the face of conditions such as large fractures, osteoporosis, bone malignancies, and genetic disorders. These challenges underscore the need for advanced therapeutic strategies that can enhance or mimic the natural regenerative processes of bone.

In recent decades, R&D&I (research, development and innovation: from basic to applied to translational science - benchtop to bedside/market) in biomaterials, scaffolds, tissue engineering, nanotechnology, and pharmaceuticals, amongst others, have revolutionized our multi-/inter-/intra-disciplinary approach to osteogenesis; de novo bone regeneration, restoration, reconstruction, replacement and repair. Biomaterials and bioactive scaffolds provide structural frameworks that support cellular activity, guiding the formation of new bone tissue. Tissue engineering strategies combine cells, growth factors, genes, drugs, and matrices to create environments conducive to regeneration, while nanotechnology has enabled the development of nanoscale interventions and localized release-controlled vehicles that enhance the delivery of therapeutic agents and improve the integration of implants with/within native tissue.

Indeed, pharmaceuticals, including osteo-inductive molecules and gene therapies, have opened new avenues for targeting the molecular pathways involved in bone repair and growth. With its promise of harnessing the body's regenerative potential, stem cell therapy has emerged as a transformative approach to treating complex bone injuries. Combinatorial therapies that integrate these advancements have shown tremendous potential, offering synergistic benefits by simultaneously addressing multiple facets of the healing process. This applies to the orthopedic and cranio-maxillo-facial skeleton.

Furthermore, the recently emerging advent of artificial intelligence (AI)-assisted technologies has enhanced our ability, as surgeons and clinicians, to diagnose, plan treatments, and monitor outcomes in bone-related conditions. AI-driven tools allow precision in imaging and modeling, enabling tailored interventions that align with our patient's unique anatomical and physiological needs. From diagnostics to treatment planning to therapy, AI and SuperAI (i.e., Trump's announced Stargate project venture) will continue reshaping the landscape of bone regeneration and repair, particularly our lives.

In this book:

- The introductory chapter establishes the foundation for understanding osteogenesis by delving into the cellular and molecular mechanisms driving bone formation, repair, and remodeling. It highlights key research, development, and innovation areas, setting the stage for the book.

- A chapter on the effects of nonsteroidal anti-inflammatory drugs (NSAIDs) on bone healing critically evaluates how these widely used medications influence bone regeneration. It challenges conventional clinical practices and emphasizes the importance of judicious treatment planning.

- A comprehensive examination of bone development and growth unpacks the genetic, hormonal, and environmental factors that shape skeletal formation and adaptation. It also explores how deviations from these processes can lead to growth and developmental disorders.

- The book includes an in-depth review of Hereditary Hemorrhagic Telangiectasia (HHT), a rare vascular disorder significantly impacting skeletal and oro-dental health. This chapter provides an overview of current knowledge, diagnostic considerations, and management strategies tailored to the unique challenges posed by HHT.

- The association between elevated non-fasting plasma total homocysteine levels and alveolar bone and tooth loss is explored in another chapter. This discussion highlights the potential for innovative diagnostic and therapeutic approaches to mitigate these effects and enhance bone health.

- The role of phyto-nanoparticles in advancing osteogenesis is another focus of this book. This chapter presents the potential of plant-derived nanomaterials in promoting bone regeneration, showcasing their versatility and bioactivity in addressing clinical challenges.

Together, these chapters and their associated bibliographies reflect the multidisciplinary nature of osteogenesis, offering a blend of fundamental science and cutting-edge advancements. They cover a broad spectrum of topics, from the impact of systemic medications to nanotechnology-driven innovations and from rare genetic disorders to novel therapeutic strategies.

Innovation in Osteogenesis Research provides an ample exploration of the dynamic field of bone regeneration, opening doors to a more comprehensive examination of the field, its status and future direction. It is designed to serve as a resource for researchers, clinicians, and students, inspiring them to push the boundaries of what is possible in bone healing, regeneration and repair. By addressing both foundational principles and novel approaches, it aims to bridge the gap between laboratory research, clinical practice and the industry (including regulatory agencies and policymakers), ultimately improving outcomes for patients (and their health care providers) worldwide.

I hope this book fosters curiosity, encourages innovation, and inspires a need to understand osteogenesis's complexities and possibilities deeply.

Bones are nature's blueprint for strength, resilience, and renewal—marvels of engineering that reveal their power to heal in every difficulty.

As scientists, we must unlock these secrets and advance their healing.

Ziyad S. Haidar, Prof. Dr.
DDS, Cert Implantol, MSc OMFS, FRCS(C), FICD, FICS, MBA, PhD,
Founder / CEO, BioMAT'X (HAiDAR R&D&I/I+D+i LABs),
Scientific Director (F-ODO) and Head of Bio-Innovation,
Centro de Investigación e Innovación Biomédica (CiiB),
Faculties of Dentistry and Medicine (Cross-Appointment),
Universidad de los Andes,
Las Condes, Santiago de Chile

Chapter 1

Introductory Chapter: Forming and Regenerating Bone – The Science of Osteogenesis, R&D&I

Ziyad S. Haidar

1. Bone development and growth

Bone development and growth, briefly, is governed by the process of osteogenesis and occur through two distinct mechanisms: intramembranous ossification and endochondral ossification [1]. Both pathways are essential for skeletal formation during embryonic development, postnatal growth, and bone repair throughout life, though they differ in their cellular pathways and developmental contexts [1, 2].

Intramembranous ossification involves the direct differentiation of mesenchymal stem cells into osteoblasts, bypassing a cartilage intermediate. This process is primarily responsible for forming flat bones, such as the skull, clavicle, and parts of the pelvis. Mesenchymal cells condense into membranous structures, differentiate into osteoblasts, and secrete the bone matrix, facilitating rapid mineralization essential for skeletal development.

Endochondral ossification, in contrast, relies on a cartilage intermediate that is gradually replaced by bone. Responsible for forming most long bones, including the limbs, spine, and ribcage, this process begins with a cartilage model that undergoes hypertrophy, vascular invasion, and subsequent replacement by bone tissue. This mechanism enables bone growth and elongation during childhood and adolescence, remodeling cartilage into mature bone.

Both ossification processes are regulated by intricate pathway signaling networks that coordinate the differentiation, proliferation, and activity of bone-forming and cartilage-forming cells [1]. Key pathways include the following:

- *Wnt/β-catenin pathway*: This pathway drives osteoblast differentiation, promoting bone matrix formation and bone mass accrual. Activation stabilizes β-catenin, which translocate to the nucleus to activate osteogenic genes. Dysregulation of Wnt signaling is associated with conditions like osteoporosis and osteosarcoma, highlighting its critical role in skeletal health.

- *Hedgehog signaling*: Crucial for chondrocyte proliferation and hypertrophy during endochondral ossification, the Hedgehog pathway governs the transition from cartilage to bone and maintains growth plate homeostasis. Sonic Hedgehog (Shh) and Indian Hedgehog (Ihh) proteins regulate gene expression to coordinate skeletal growth and patterning.

- *Bone morphogenetic proteins (BMPs) and TGF-β signaling*: BMPs, particularly BMP-2 and BMP-7 (*also referred to as OP-1 or osteogenic protein-1*), stimulate osteoblast activity and extracellular matrix production, playing key roles in bone grafts and fracture healing. TGF-β signaling influences both osteoblasts and osteoclasts, regulating progenitor cell commitment to the osteoblastic lineage and coordinating bone remodeling and mineralization.

These pathways [1, 2] ensure that bone development and remodeling respond appropriately to developmental, mechanical, and metabolic demands. Disruptions in these closely regulated processes can result in developmental disorders, impaired bone healing, or conditions such as osteoporosis and skeletal dysplasia [3]. Henceforth, advances in understanding these mechanisms have not only deepened insights into bone biology but have also driven the development of innovative therapies for enhancing osteogenesis, bone regeneration, and treating skeletal disorders.

2. Challenges in bone healing

As aforementioned, bone possesses a remarkable ability to regenerate, but this process can be disrupted under certain conditions, leading to delayed or failed healing. These disruptions present significant clinical challenges, particularly in cases involving critical-sized defects, non-union fractures, osteoporosis, and bone infections, each requiring specialized therapeutic approaches [1–3]. Critical-sized defects are large bone injuries that cannot heal naturally within a patient's lifetime, often resulting from traumatic injuries or congenital deformities [3, 4]. The main challenge in treating these defects is providing structural stability while promoting biological repair [3]. Traditional bone grafts, such as autografts, allografts, and xenografts, have limitations, including donor site morbidity, limited availability, and potential immune responses [3–5]. This has driven the development of synthetic biomaterials designed to mimic the mechanical properties and osteoinductive capacity of natural bone [3–8]. Non-union fractures occur when a bone fails to heal after an extended period, often due to poor vascular supply, infection, or systemic conditions like diabetes [6–8]. Addressing these fractures requires advanced therapies to stimulate the healing process, including the use of bone morphogenetic proteins (BMPs), stem cell-based treatments, and biocompatible scaffolds that promote vascularization and osteogenesis [8]. Osteoporosis, which is characterized by reduced bone mass and deteriorating bone structure, complicates bone healing, particularly in the elderly [4, 7, 8]. Healing in osteoporotic patients is hindered by poor bone quality and reduced osteoblast activity, leading to heightened osteoclast-mediated resorption [7, 8]. Treatments aim to improve bone density and enhance osteogenesis, with agents such as bisphosphonates, selective estrogen receptor modulators (SERMs), and anabolic therapies like parathyroid hormone (PTH) analogs. Emerging therapies, including monoclonal antibodies targeting osteoclast activity and novel approaches stimulating bone formation via pathways like Wnt signaling, offer new potential for improving healing outcomes [3–8]. Bone infections, or osteomyelitis, are particularly challenging due to the need to both eradicate infection and restore bone integrity [9]. Chronic infections can disrupt bone remodeling, leading to significant bone loss [10]. Treatment typically involves a combination of surgical debridement, antibiotic therapy, and bone reconstruction, with innovative drug delivery systems, such as antibiotic-laden scaffolds and release-controlled core-shell nano-capsules loaded with recombinant osteogenic proteins (*reader is invited to visit our lab's publications*), offering promising solutions for localized infection control while supporting bone regeneration [10, 11]. Furthermore, patient-specific factors such as age, nutritional deficiencies, smoking, and comorbid conditions like diabetes or vascular diseases can complicate bone healing, requiring personalized treatment strategies to address both systemic and local barriers to repair.

3. Innovative approaches to overcome bone healing challenges

To recap, addressing the accruing challenges of bone healing has fueled the design, development, and translation of emerging technologies and therapies tailored to enhance biological healing, bridge critical defects, and promote osteogenesis in non-union fractures [9, 10]. These innovations also aim to improve healing in osteoporotic patients and combat infections such as osteomyelitis. By integrating tissue engineering, regenerative medicine, and biotechnology, these strategies offer new solutions to overcome traditional barriers in bone repair, focusing on regeneration, osteogenesis, and tissue integrity **Figure 1** [9–11].

4. Biological enhancements

Biological therapies using growth factors like BMPs and VEGF show promise in accelerating bone regeneration, repair, restoration, and healing. As previously indicated, BMPs promote osteogenesis via stimulating mesenchymal stem cell differentiation into osteoblasts, while VEGF encourages the formation of new blood vessels, improving nutrient supply to healing bone [2, 4, 6, 7]. Stem cell-based therapies,

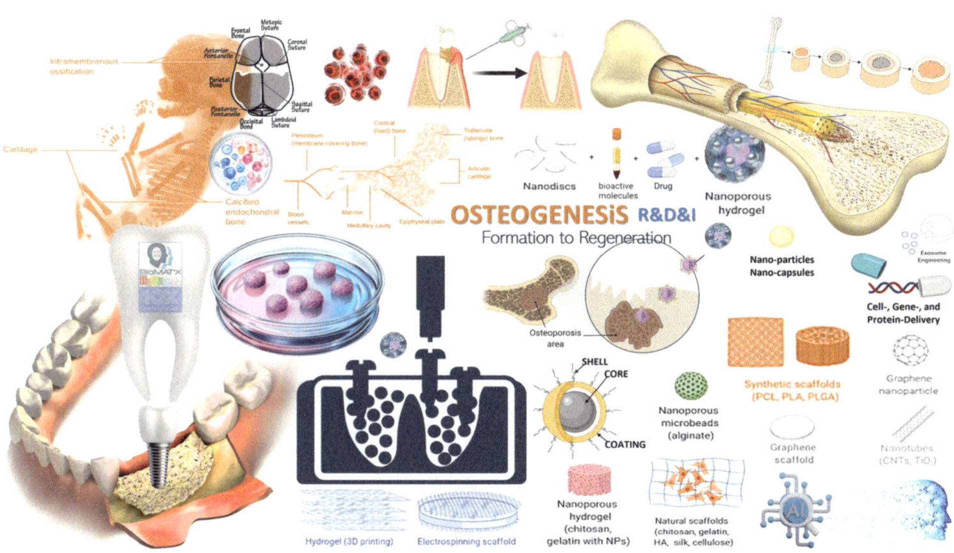

Figure 1.
Innovations in osteogenesis: *From natural bone development and repair to advanced R&D&I tools and strategies for enhanced and accelerated bone regeneration, utilizing biomaterials, nanotechnology, pharmaceuticals, tissue engineering, and AI-assisted technologies.*

particularly using mesenchymal stromal/stem cells (MSCs), are key to enhancing and/or promoting tissue regeneration. MSCs not only differentiate into osteoblasts but also release signals that help improve the local healing environment and stimulate vascularization, critical for large or compromised bone structures [5, 10].

5. Engineered materials

Engineered biomaterials are designed to overcome the limitations of traditional bone grafts, offering materials that mimic the mechanical and biological properties of natural bone [2–4, 6]. These include 3D-printed scaffolds, bioactive glass, and composite materials, which provide structural support while encouraging osteogenesis. Further, by functionalizing these materials with bioactive molecules or nanoparticles, their regenerative potential is further enhanced (smart/intelligent biomaterials). For example, scaffolds loaded with BMPs release these factors at the injury site, promoting bone formation, locally. Additionally, materials such as hydroxyapatite and collagen improve biocompatibility and help implants integrate better with surrounding tissue, reducing the risk of implant failure [3, 6, 8, 9].

6. Combination therapies

Combining biomaterials with biological agents and bioactive pharmacological treatments provides a comprehensive approach to bone healing and repair. This strategy addresses the biological, structural, and microbial aspects of healing simultaneously [1, 2, 6, 9]. Scaffolds can be loaded with both BMPs and antibiotics, offering structural support and antimicrobial protection, which is particularly important in cases of osteomyelitis. Combining stem cell therapies with engineered biomaterials enhances the survival, integration, and differentiation of stem cells at the injury and/or surgical site. This integrated combinatorial approach creates a more conducive healing environment, improving both the efficacy and predictability of bone regeneration and repair interventions.

7. Regenerative medicine and dentistry – *A perspective*

Regenerative medicine and dentistry are poised to revolutionize tissue healing and restoration by harnessing the natural healing abilities. Through advancements in tissue engineering, biomaterials, nanobiotechnology, pharmaceuticals, and cellular therapies, the treatment of complex orthopedic bone, cranio-oro-maxillo-facial, and dental disorders is entering a new era. These innovations promise to redefine therapeutic options, offering more effective treatments and improved patient outcomes.

Whilst the transition from pre-clinical research to clinical application in regenerative therapies is full of potential, challenges persist. Some of the key hurdles include regulatory approval, patient safety, and meeting efficacy standards. Regulatory frameworks must evolve alongside rapid technological advancements, while scalable production methods are crucial for widespread clinical use [12]. On the other hand, biomanufacturing techniques including bioreactors and automated cell culture systems are facilitating the efficient production of cell-based therapies, biomaterials, and bioactive molecules.

In regenerative dentistry, significant strides are being made in addressing dental and periodontal tissue damage. Techniques like guided tissue regeneration (GTR) promote the regeneration of bone and ligaments, while bioactive-coated dental implants are enhancing treatment outcomes. Additionally, signaling molecules are increasing the effectiveness of regenerative procedures in periodontitis and stabilizing dental implants [5, 6, 9].

That said, the future of regenerative therapies lies in personalized treatments, 3D bioprinting, and advanced drug delivery systems. 3D-printed patient-specific implants, designed to mimic the biological and mechanical properties of native tissues, demonstrate great promise in treating complex defects. Furthermore, immunomodulation strategies, such as stem cell homing, are simplifying therapies by reducing reliance on external cells, and when combined with nanotechnology, it allows for highly targeted, localized drug delivery [5, 6, 9]. Pharmaceutical innovations, including sclerostin inhibitors, PTH analogs, and bisphosphonates, are advancing the potential of regenerative medicine, particularly for bone-related conditions. These therapies, paired with novel drug delivery systems like nanocarriers, aim to regulate osteogenesis and promote bone regeneration at the molecular level. Herein, nanotechnology is, in parallel, contributing to transforming bone regeneration by enabling the manipulation of materials at the molecular level. Nanomaterials, such as titanium dioxide and carbon nanotubes, enhance bioactivity and accelerate healing. Gold and silver nanoparticles, as well as natural polymer-based nano-capsules, possess osteogenic properties, and bioresorbable nanomaterials enable effective local drug delivery to injury sites [2, 10, 11]. Today, digital technologies are enhancing precision and accessibility in regenerative medicine and dentistry. While telemedicine and tele-dentistry enable remote consultations, advanced imaging systems, including cone-beam computed tomography (CBCT) and augmented reality, are improving surgical planning and execution. More so, AI-driven tools, predictive models, and automated image analysis help refine interventions, making care more personalized and precise [12, 13]. Finally, wearable health devices and smart implants help our patients monitor healing in real-time, promoting adaptive rehabilitation, timely feedback, and early intervention [8, 10]. As regenerative medicine progresses, the challenging regulatory frameworks, previously highlighted, can be expected to adapt to ensure safety, efficacy, and accessibility. Balancing innovation with stringent safety standards is essential for widespread translation and adoption. Ethical considerations surrounding gene editing, stem cell therapies, and AI-powered diagnostics are being addressed, along with safeguarding patient privacy. Transparency in research, development, and innovation will be key to fostering trust, attracting funding, and advancing impact on our patients.

8. The road ahead

Looking ahead, the intersection of regenerative medicine, biotechnology, and artificial intelligence offers immense potential for transforming the landscape of bone and dental regeneration [14, 15]. The integration of personalized medicine, nanotechnology, and innovative drug delivery systems promises to deliver unprecedented advances in patient care [15]. However, to realize the full potential of these innovations, interdisciplinary collaborations among researchers, clinicians, and regulatory bodies will be essential [15]. By aligning cutting-edge scientific breakthroughs with ethical principles and regulatory frameworks, the promise of regenerative medicine and dentistry can be fully realized [14, 15]. In conclusion, osteogenic regenerative medicine and dentistry are entering an exciting era of innovation, with the potential to transform how we approach bone and its health. The future is bright, with advancements in personalized treatments, nanotechnology, digital medicine, stem cell therapies, and sustainable biomaterials [14, 15] paving the way for more effective, accessible, and tailored solutions for patients. By addressing the challenges ahead with a balanced approach, we can look forward to a future where regenerative medicine and dentistry deliver groundbreaking osteogenic solutions that significantly improve patient (as well as surgeon and/or health care provider) outcomes and quality of life.

Acknowledgements

This work was supported by operating grants provided to the HAiDAR R&D&I LAB/BioMAT'X (Laboratorio de Biomateriales, Farmacéuticos y Bioingeniería de Tejidos Cráneo Máxilo-Facial), member of CiiB (Centro de Investigación e Innovación Biomédica), Faculties of Medicine and Dentistry, Universidad de los Andes, Santiago de Chile, through the ANID-NAM (Agencia Nacional de Investigación y Desarrollo, Chile, and National Academy of Medicine, USA), Grant código # NAM21I0022 (2020–2022), CORFO Crea y Valida I + D + i, Grant código # 21CVC2-183649 (2021–2023), CORFO Crea y Valida -Proyecto de I + D + i Colaborativo –Reactívate," Grant código # 22CVC2-218196 (2022–2024), and FONDEF Concurso IDEA de I + D, ANID, Grant código # ID22I10215 (2022–2024).

Author's note

This introductory chapter was prepared with the assistance of OpenAI tools such as Trinka AI for specific purposes of language and grammar refinement. Herein, all content has been reviewed and edited, and the final manuscript was polished by the author to ensure accuracy, integrity, relevance, and clarity to the readers.

Conflict of interest

The author declares no conflict of interest.

DOI: http://dx.doi.org/10.5772/intechopen.1009273

Author details

Ziyad S. Haidar
BioMAT'X (HAiDAR LAB) R&D&I, Biomedical Research and Innovation Center (CiiB), Faculties of Medicine and Dentistry, University of the Andes, Las Condes, Santiago, Chile

*Address all correspondence to: zhaidar@uandes.cl; zhaidar78@gmail.com

References

[1] Dimitriou R, Jones E, McGonagle D, Giannoudis PV. Bone regeneration: Current concepts and future directions. BMC Medicine. 2011;**9**(1):66. DOI: 10.1186/1741-7015-9-66

[2] Oryan A, Alidadi S, Moshiri A, Maffulli N. Bone regenerative medicine: Classic options, novel strategies, and future directions. Journal of Orthopaedic Surgery and Research. 2014;**9**:18. DOI: 10.1186/1749-799X-9-18

[3] Rezwan K, Chen QZ, Blaker JJ, Boccaccini AR. Biodegradable and bioactive porous polymer/inorganic composite scaffolds for bone tissue engineering. Biomaterials. 2006;**27**(18):3413-3431. DOI: 10.1016/j.biomaterials.2006.01.039

[4] Hench LL, Polak JM. Third-generation biomedical materials. Science. 2002;**295**(5557):1014-1017. DOI: 10.1126/science.1067404

[5] Chim H, Schantz JT. New frontiers in calvarial reconstruction: Integrating computer-assisted design and tissue engineering in cranioplasty. Plastic and Reconstructive Surgery. 2005;**116**(6):1726-1741. DOI: 10.1097/01.prs.0000182386.78775.cd

[6] Fröhlich M, Grayson WL, Wan LQ, Marolt D, Drobnic M, Vunjak-Novakovic G. Tissue engineered bone grafts: Biological requirements, tissue culture and clinical relevance. Current Stem Cell Research and Therapy. 2008;**3**(4):254-264. DOI: 10.2174/157488808786733962

[7] Drosse I, Volkmer E, Capanna R, De Biase P, Schieker M. Tissue engineering for bone defect healing: An update on a multi-component approach. Injury. 2008;**39**(Suppl 2):S9-S20. DOI: 10.1016/S0020-1383(08)70011-1

[8] Einhorn TA, Gerstenfeld LC. Fracture healing: Mechanisms and interventions. Nature Reviews Rheumatology. 2015;**11**(1):45-54. DOI: 10.1038/nrrheum.2014.164

[9] Li D, Zhang D, Yuan Q, Liu L, Li H, Xiong L, et al. In vitro and in vivo assessment of the effect of biodegradable magnesium alloys on osteogenesis. Acta Biomaterialia. 2022;**141**:454-465. DOI: 10.1016/j.actbio.2021.12.032. Epub 2021 Dec 28

[10] Bauso LV, La Fauci V, Longo C, Calabrese G. Bone tissue engineering and nanotechnology: A promising combination for bone regeneration. Biology (Basel). 2024;**13**(4):237. DOI: 10.3390/biology13040237

[11] Saiz E, Zimmermann EA, Lee JS, Wegst UG, Tomsia AP. Perspectives on the role of nanotechnology in bone tissue engineering. Dental Materials. 2013;**29**(1):103-115. DOI: 10.1016/j.dental.2012.08.001. Epub 2012 Aug 14

[12] Topol EJ. High-performance medicine: The convergence of human and artificial intelligence. Nature Medicine. 2019;**25**(1):44-56. DOI: 10.1038/s41591-018-0300-7

[13] Hamet P, Tremblay J. Artificial intelligence in medicine. Metabolism. 2017;**69**:S36-S40. DOI: 10.1016/j.metabol.2017.01.011

[14] Muñoz F, Haidar ZS, Puigdollers A, Guerra I, Padilla MC, Ortega N, et al. A novel

Chilean salmon fish backbone-based nanoHydroxyApatite functional biomaterial for potential use in bone tissue engineering. Frontiers in Medicine (Lausanne). 2024;**11**:1330482. DOI: 10.3389/fmed.2024.1330482

[15] Jawadi Z, Yang C, Haidar ZS, Santa Maria PL, Massa S. Bio-inspired muco-adhesive polymers for drug delivery applications. Polymers (Basel). 2022;**14**(24):5459. DOI: 10.3390/polym14245459

Chapter 2

NSAIDs Effect on Bone Healing

Rana Muhammad Zeeshan

Abstract

The extensive use of non-steroidal anti-inflammatory drugs (NSAIDs) for the treatment of severe pain associated with bone fractures raises concerns regarding their impact on fracture healing. While NSAIDs are favored for their anti-inflammatory properties, long-term administration has been associated with adverse effects on fracture healing. Despite the recognized risks, conflicting information exists regarding the effects of NSAIDs on fracture healing. Fracture healing is a complex process involving mechanisms of repair, including direct and indirect bone healing pathways. The inflammatory phase plays a crucial role in initiating the healing, with immune cells secreting cytokines and growth factors essential for healing. Prostaglandins, synthesized by COX enzymes, are key mediators, exerting stimulatory effects on bone formation and resorption. However, NSAIDs inhibit prostaglandin synthesis by blocking COX activity, disrupting the fracture-healing process. NSAIDs also have an inhibitory effect on the differentiation of chondrocytes into mature hypertrophied chondrocytes, crucial for endochondral ossification. Collagen X, expressed by hypertrophied chondrocytes, serves as a vital marker of fracture healing and has been implicated in the successful union of fractures. A comprehensive understanding of the interplay between NSAIDs, prostaglandins, and fracture healing mechanisms is essential for optimizing treatment strategies and minimizing adverse outcomes in patients with bone fractures.

Keywords: fracture healing, prostaglandins, cartilaginous callus, bone callus, NSAIDs, cyclooxygenase enzyme, mature hypertrophied chondrocytes, collagen type X

1. Introduction

Bone fractures are a public health issue affecting humans globally. In 2019, 178 million new fracture cases were seen globally, with an increase of 33.4%, and 455 million cases of acute or long-term symptoms of fracture were registered, which has increased to 70.1% since 1990. The chief complaint about bone fracture is chronic severe pain that results from damage to somatosensory nerve terminals, which innervates bones and muscles. For the treatment of severe pain, most used analgesics are non-steroidal anti-inflammatory drugs (NSAIDs). NSAIDs are preferred over different analgesics in fracture healing due to their anti-inflammatory effect in addition to pain relieving. However, long-term administration of NSAIDs is related to increased rates of delayed union, malunion, and non-union. Administration of NSAIDs can cause malunion, non-union, and delayed fracture healing due to inhibitory effects on cyclooxygenase-2 (COX-2) enzyme, which is essential for the synthesis of prostaglandins and interferes in the inflammatory phase of healing, which leads to an inhibitory effect on fracture healing [1–6].

Controversial information exists regarding the effects of NSAIDs on the fracture healing process; at the same time, there is a lack of comparative information about fracture healing with the intake of non-selective COX and selective COX-2 inhibitors and localization of collagen X expressed by hypertrophied chondrocytes in the healing fracture.

2. Fracture healing

2.1 Definition

The process of fracture healing occurs through a regenerative biological process that heals the loss of mechanical continuity in a bone resulting from the pathological mobility between the broken ends of a bone [7].

2.2 Factors that affect bone healing

The following factors play a vital role in bone healing process:

1. Delayed bone healing is seen in nutritional deficits and metabolic disorders, especially in diabetes mellitus.

2. Parathyroid hormones have a vital role in bone healing as they stimulate the proliferation and differentiation of osteoblasts and osteoclasts.

3. Aging

4. Infection of the fracture site delays the healing process [8].

2.3 Mechanisms of repair

The mechanism of fracture repair is divided into two categories, which are direct (primary) and indirect (secondary) bone healing, depending on differences in local motion between the fracture fragments.

2.3.1 Direct bone healing

In direct fracture healing, the cortex tries to bridge the continuity between the fracture fragments by regeneration, and this occurs only when the rigid internal fixation is established between fracture fragments. Fractured ends heal without the formation of a callus [9].

Direct healing of fractures exists through two processes: contact healing and gap healing. In both these processes, lamellar bone structure is formed between the fractured ends [10].

Contact healing occurs when the gap is less than 0.01 mm between fractured ends, and there is less than 2% of interfragmentary strain. In this process of contact healing at the ends of the osteons, cutting cones are formed, and the tips of these cutting cones cross the fracture line. These tips have osteoclasts that generate longitudinal cavities. These cavities are filled by new bone synthesized by osteoblasts, resulting in bony union and restoration of Haversian systems. The Haversian systems help in carrying osteoblasts to enter the area through blood vessels. In the end, bridging osteons mature into lamellar bone, leading to fracture healing without a callus formation [11].

In the gap healing process, the gap between fractured ends must be less than 800 μm between fractured fragments. The bone union and Haversian remodeling do not occur simultaneously. At the fracture site, a large amount of lamellar bone is present running perpendicular to the long axis, and this needs secondary reconstruction of osteonal tissue. Longitudinal revascularized osteons replace the primary bone structure and carry osteoprogenitor cells that differentiate into osteoblasts, which produce lamellar bone on each surface of the gap. This newly formed lamellar bone is laid down perpendicular to the long axis and is very weak in strength, which is then strengthened by Haversian remodeling without the formation of callus [11].

2.3.2 Indirect bone healing

Indirect fracture healing occurs due to the involvement of the periosteum and soft tissues surrounding the fracture site. This response is improved by restricted fracture fragment movement and is repressed by rigid fixation. This type of fracture healing comprises two processes: intramembranous and endochondral bone formation. Endochondral bone formation begins in a mechanically less stable region, which is near the fracture site outside the periosteum, whereas internal to the periosteum, a hard callus is formed by intramembranous ossification [12, 13].

2.4 Phases of fracture healing

The process of fracture healing comprises distinct phases, starting with an initial anabolic phase, in which local tissue size increases through inflammation and hematoma is formed (**Figure 1**). After hematoma formation, the inflammatory phase occurs, followed by the development of soft and hard callus, ultimately leading to bone remodeling [10].

2.4.1 Hematoma formation

The impact force of trauma causing the fracture disturbs the normal bone structure with disruption of blood vessels at the site of contact, consequently leading to hematoma formation. The hematoma produced by vascular damage contains immune cells that migrate from the circulation and bone marrow to the injury site [15, 16].

2.4.2 Inflammatory phase

Hematoma formation triggers the early inflammatory phase, the role of which is most vital in initiating the process of the healing cascade. Inflammatory cells exert chemotactic effects and further recruit inflammatory and mesenchymal cells that are essential for fracture healing. These cells play a significant role in stimulating angiogenesis and extracellular matrix synthesis.

Inflammatory cells produce cytokines that affect fracture healing as the pro-inflammatory molecule interleukin 1(IL1) secreted by macrophages regulates the

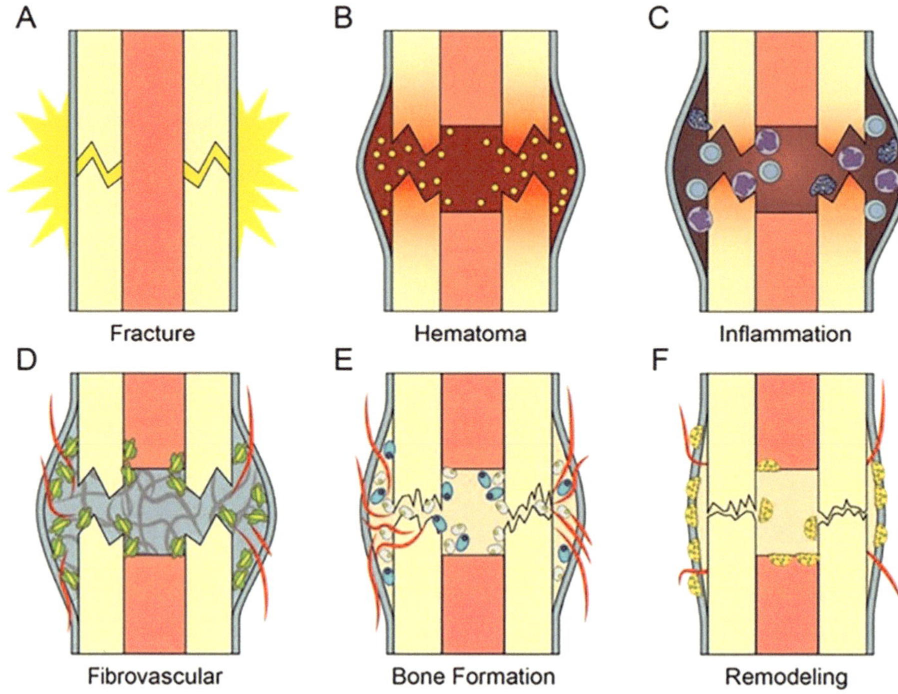

Figure 1.
Different phases of fracture healing [14].

expression of cyclooxygenases (COX1 and COX2) enzymes which produce prostaglandins. During the inflammatory phase of fracture healing, inflammatory cells secrete several important growth factors including fibroblast growth factors (FGF), transforming growth factor-beta (TGF-beta), and platelet-derived growth factor (PDGF) which help and facilitate the process of fracture healing.

These factors after their secretion initiate the repair process as they promote and facilitate the stem cell proliferation and differentiation that results at the beginning of the formation of the fracture callus. Other principal factors released include tumor necrosis factor alpha, bone morphogenic protein, interleukin 6, interleukin 17F, and interleukin 23 [10, 14, 17].

2.4.3 Formation of cartilaginous callus

The next phase of fracture healing is the formation of a soft callus, also called cartilaginous callus. On a cellular level, chondrocytes and fibrocytes are predominant in the healing tissue. These cells form a soft callus (semi-solid) that provides mechanical support to the fracture. This soft callus acts as a stencil for the bony callus. Initially, the cartilaginous callus is avascular, but when the cartilaginous tissue is replaced by woven bone, vasculogenesis occurs, which results in vascular invasion of the healing tissue. The mesenchymal stem cells differentiate into chondrocytes in the central fracture area, leading to the formation of the soft callus and different growth factors expressed in soft callus including TGF-α2, PDGF, IGF-1, and BMPs. These growth factors stimulate the proliferation and differentiation of chondrocytes. The increased population of chondrocytes stabilizes the fracture zone [18, 19].

2.4.4 Formation of bony callus

The bony callus formation phase occurs after cartilaginous callus formation; chondrocytes present in the healing zone start to proliferate and mature to become hypertrophic. Chondrocytes, during the initial phase of bony callus formation, undergo a series of differentiation, leading to the formation of hypertrophic chondrocytes. This leads to an increase in the synthesis of collagen X that accumulates inside the extracellular matrix.

Mature hypertrophied chondrocytes are present adjacent to the tidemark within the deep layer of articular cartilage. COLX is a crucial factor in the successful union of fractures in the tissues going under endochondral ossification. The hypertrophic chondrocytes secrete angiogenic factors necessary for osteoclast and osteoblast recruitment, which is an essential step in bone formation.

Osteoclast acts to reabsorb the calcified matrix made by the hypertrophic chondrocytes whereas definitive bone formation is done by osteoblasts. Additional mesenchymal progenitor cells start to recruit and differentiate into osteoblasts, as chondrocytes undergo apoptosis, thus leading to the mineralization of the callus. This mineralized callus is called bony callus, which is composed of a thin layer of bone tissue around the periphery of soft callus [20–23].

2.4.5 Angiogenesis and bone remodeling

New blood vessels continue to form with the action of vascular endothelial growth factor (VEGF). In the later phase, the bony callus grows through the action of osteoblasts, and bone resorption occurs by osteoclasts to reshape the callus. Both osteoblastic bone formation and osteoclastic bone resorption occur side by side, resulting in the regeneration of the original bone tissue architecture, which contains the outer cortical bone and inner trabeculae arrangement with a central space called the medullary cavity which contains the bone marrow [24].

2.5 Role of inflammatory cells in fracture healing

The key step in fracture healing is the inflammatory phase, as several immune cells are recruited to the injury site, which include neutrophils, platelets, and macrophages, and they are activated by cytokines. As immune cells invade the hematoma, they secrete cytokines and growth factors that help recruit mesenchymal cells. The growth factors (FGF, PDGF, TGFb, and FGF) and cytokines (IL-1, IL-6, and tumor necrosis factor (TNF)), which are released by inflammatory cells, influence prostaglandin production in the presence of pro-inflammatory stimuli. These cytokine and growth factors especially prostaglandins are produced by osteoblasts abundantly in fracture callus following fracture injury during the first 2 weeks [25, 26].

To understand the role of prostaglandins in bone healing process, we must know about their synthesis, mode of action, and how their inhibition affects the healing cascade in inflammatory process, which is discussed in the next section.

3. Prostaglandins: a key mediator

During the fracture healing process, prostaglandins are important lipid mediators that are synthesized by enzymes cyclooxygenase (COX-1 or COX-2) from arachidonic acid. These enzymes regulate inflammation and help in the synthesis of prostaglandins as they catalyze the early enzymatic stages. Prostaglandins are potent stimulators of bone formation as well as bone resorption. Their increased production stimulates vascular changes, chondrocyte differentiation, proliferation of osteogenic cells, and bone resorption in response to fracture. Prostaglandins increase collagen X expression with the help of bone morphogenetic protein 4 and growth/differentiation factor 5, which enhances chondrocyte growth and differentiation [27–30].

3.1 Classification of prostaglandins

Prostaglandins belong to the family of eicosanoids which are composed of eicosa-(20-carbon) polyenoic fatty acids. Classes of eicosanoids comprise the prostanoid, leukotrienes (LTs), and lipoxins (LXs). Prostanoids include prostaglandins (PGs), prostacyclins (PGIs), and thromboxanes (TXs). There are four principal bioactive prostaglandins synthesized *in vivo*, which are prostaglandin (PG) E2 (PGE2), prostacyclin (PGI2), prostaglandin D2 (PGD2), and prostaglandin F2α (PGF2α) [31, 32].

3.2 Biosynthesis of prostaglandins

Prostaglandins are biosynthesized starting from the release of arachidonic acid from the plasma membrane phospholipids catalyzed by activated phospholipase A2 (**Figure 2**). Arachidonic acid is then converted to PGH2 by enzymes, cyclooxygenase, and peroxidase activities of PGH synthase, which is known as cyclooxygenase (COX) [34].

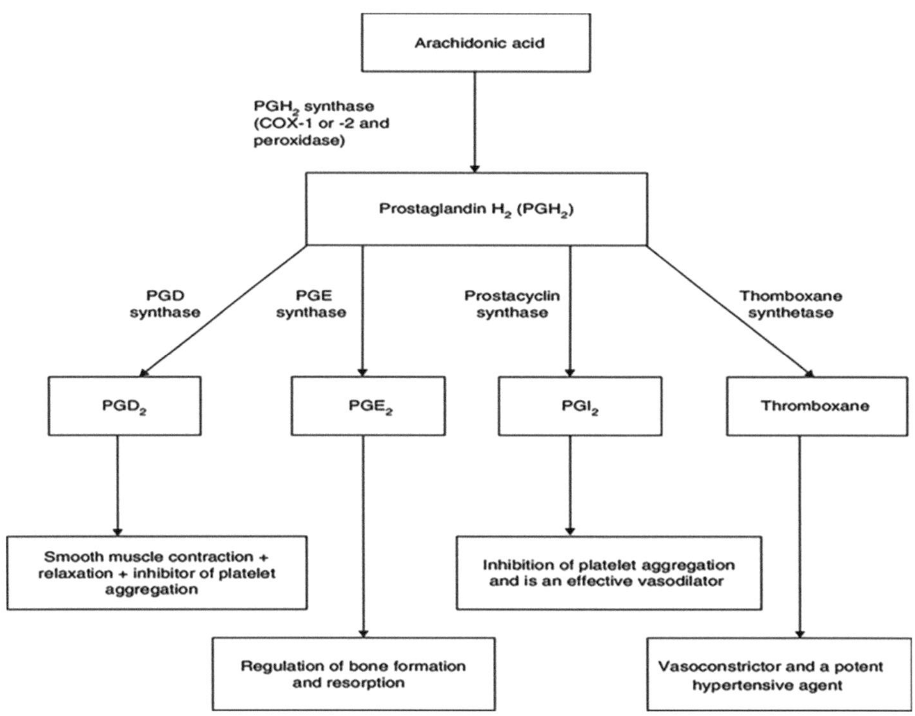

Figure 2.
Biosynthetic pathways of prostaglandins with their functions [33].

PGE2 is formed by the action of enzyme PGE synthase, PGD synthase acts to form PGD2, which is present in brain and mast cells, and prostaglandin F2α is produced by the enzyme Prostaglandin F (PGF) synthase present in the uterus. Thromboxane synthases present in platelets and macrophages act to produce thromboxane A2 and thromboxane B2, whereas prostacyclin synthase is found in endothelial cells, and prostacyclin synthase produces prostacyclin PGI2 [35].

3.2.1 Action of cyclooxygenase enzymes

Cyclooxygenase (COX) enzyme catalyzes the first two steps in the formation of prostaglandins. There are two main COX isoforms, COX-1 and COX-2. These two enzymes are the main targets of the commonly used NSAIDs, and they demonstrate the role of these enzymes in pain, fever, inflammation, and tumorigenesis. COX-1 is involved functionally in normal physiological functions, and COX-2 acts as an immediately acting agent produced rapidly induced by growth factors, oncogenes, carcinogens, and tumor-related substances [36, 37].

3.3 Functions of prostaglandins E2

Prostaglandins E2 has extensive spectrum actions on various organs, including inflammation, fracture healing, physiological bone formation, embryo implantation, vasodilation, and induction of labor. There are four G protein-coupled receptor subtypes, EP1R–EP4R (E-prostanoid receptor), which mediate the pharmacological activities of PGE2 [38].

3.3.1 Role in bone metabolism

Prostaglandin E2 plays either a stimulatory or an inhibitory role in bone metabolism, depending on the physiological or pathological conditions. Bone formation occurs in response to mechanical forces and bone fracture healing, whereas PGE2-mediated resorption contributes to bone loss in inflammatory diseases and prolonged immobilization. The binding of PGE2 to E-prostanoid receptor 2 appears to stimulate bone formation as it strongly acts on the osteoblastic lineage and stimulates bone formation, whereas PGE2 binding to E-prostanoid receptor 4 results in bone resorption due to the stimulation of osteoclast differentiation by cytokines and upregulation of the nuclear factor k-B ligand-receptor expression resulting in inhibition of osteoprotegerin expression in osteoblastic cells [39, 40].

3.4 Inhibition of prostaglandins synthesis

Prostaglandin synthesis is inhibited by the action of non-steroidal anti-inflammatory drugs (NSAIDs) as they inhibit the cyclooxygenase (COX) enzyme, which controls the biosynthesis of prostaglandins and thromboxane. The synthesis of PGE2 is inhibited by widely used non-steroidal anti-inflammatory drugs given in the treatment of inflammation, pain, and fever by blocking COX activity. Prostaglandins are essential for normal bone turnover and fracture healing. Therefore, the use of NSAIDs may affect bone healing by inhibiting the maturation of the callus [41–43].

So, the question here is why NSAIDs are still being administered in patients suffering from musculoskeletal conditions, especially in fracture healing. To answer this question, firstly, we need to understand NSAIDs and their benefits, discussed in the next section.

4. NSAIDs: most used analgesic drug

Non-steroidal anti-inflammatory drugs (NSAIDs) are the most common analgesics used for treating acute and chronic musculoskeletal disorders including traumas. NSAIDs decrease the increased pain threshold that is related to inflammation instead of elevating the normal pain threshold; therefore, its antinociceptive action is described as antihyperalgesic rather than analgesic [44, 45].

4.1 Classification of NSAIDs

4.1.1 Based on structure and selectivity

NSAIDs are divided into groups which are based on the chemical structure and their selectivity as non-selective, which are acetylated salicylates commonly known as aspirin, non-acetylated salicylates, acetic acids, propionic acids, which comprises

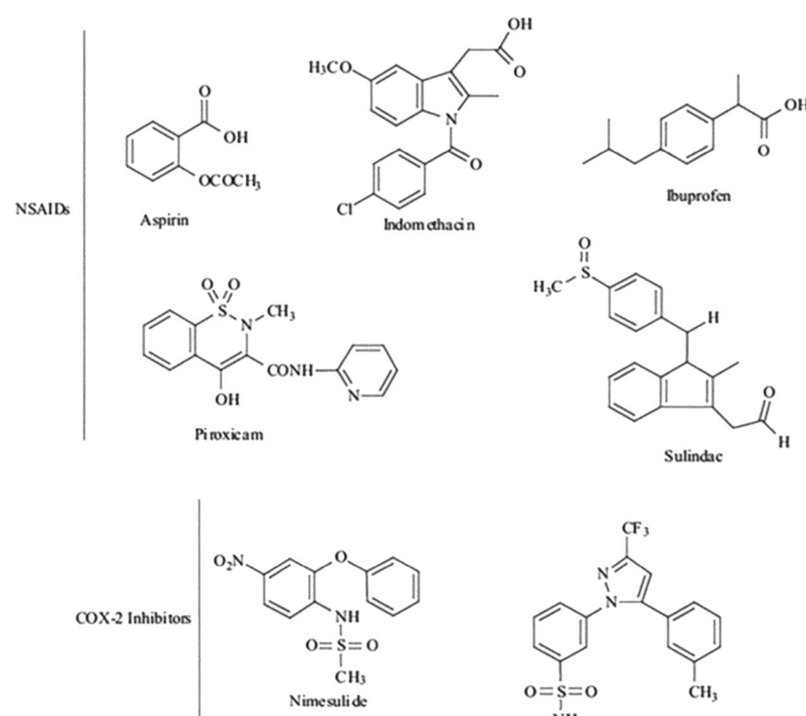

Figure 3.
Chemical structure of commonly used NSAIDs [46].

Group	Drugs	Dosage	Side effects
Salicylic acid derivates	Acetylsalicylic acid (aspirin) Sodium salicylate Diflunisal Sulfasalazine Olsalazine	1200-1500 mg (8 hourly) 1200-1500 mg (8 hourly) 500 mg (12 hourly) 2–3 g daily 500 mg (12 hourly)	Gastric upset, gastric, and duodenal ulcers Gastric upset, gastric, and duodenal ulcers Gastric upset, dry mouth, and drowsiness Nausea, vomiting, headache, and rash Gastric upset, nausea, and bloating
Para-aminophenol derivatives	Acetaminophen	500 mg (6 hourly)	Hepatic toxicity
Indol and indene acetic acid	Indomethacin Sulindac Etodolac	50-70 mg (8 hourly) 200 mg (12 hourly) 200-300 mg (6 hourly)	Pancreatitis, headache, dizziness, confusion, and depression Stevens–Johnson epidermal necrolysis syndrome, thrombocytopenia, agranulocytosis, and nephrotic syndrome Heartburn, bloody vomiting, and diarrhea
Heteroaryl acetic acid	Ibuprofen Neproxen Flurbiprofen Ketoprofen Fenoprofen Oxaprozin	600 mg (6 hourly) 375 mg (12 hourly) 300 mg (6 hourly) 70 mg (6 hourly) 600 mg (6 hourly) 1200-1800 mg (6 hourly)	Headache, dizziness, drowsiness, fatigue, and restless sleep Tinitus, Itching of skin Dizziness, rash, and tinnitus Dizziness, rash, and tinnitus Acidity, headache, and heartburn Dizziness, wheezing, and blurred vision
Anthranilic acid (fenemates)	Mefenamic acid Meclofenamic acid	500 mg daily initially, then 250 mg (6 hourly) 500 mg daily initially, then 250 mg (6 hourly)	Diarrhea, nausea, and hypertension Abdominal pain, nausea, and rash
Enolic acid derivatives (oxicams)	Piroxicam Tenoxicam Meloxicam	20 mg (6 hourly) 20 mg daily 10 mg daily	Black tarry stools, decreased urination, and severe stomach pain Headache, nausea, vomiting, and epigastric pain Headache, dizziness, and abdominal pain

Table 1.
Classification of NSAIDs according to structure.

naproxen, ibuprofen, diclofenac, and indomethacin, enolic acids, anthranilic acids (mefenamic acid), naphthylalanine, and selective COX-2 inhibitors (**Figure 3**; **Table 1**) [47].

4.1.2 Based on COX enzyme inhibition

Based on their effect on cyclooxygenase enzymes (COX-1 and COX-2), NSAIDs are classified as COX-1 selective, non-selective, COX-2 preferential, and COX-2 selective [48].

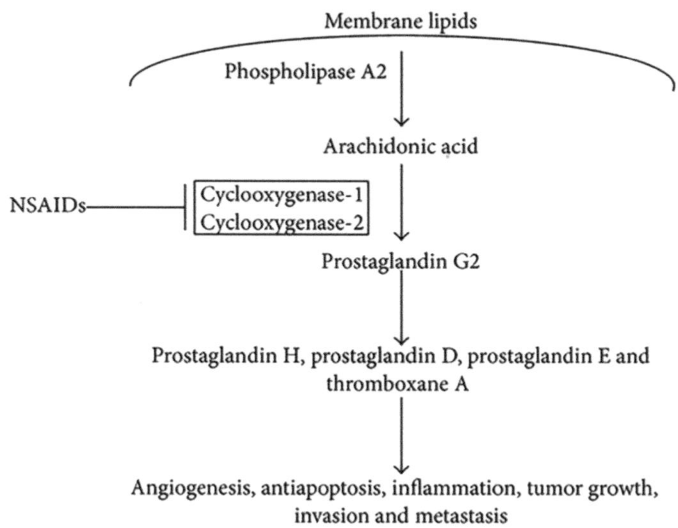

Figure 4.
Schematic of the mechanism of action of NSAIDs [49].

4.2 Function of NSAIDs

The main function of NSAIDs is to halt the synthesis and action of important inflammatory mediators which are synthesized during inflammation. These mediators include prostaglandins, coagulation cascade-derived peptides, interleukins (IL-2 and IL-6), and tumor necrosis factor (TNF). In the synthesis of prostaglandins, COX-1 and COX-2 are the rate-limiting enzymes that convert arachidonic acid into prostaglandins (**Figure 4**). So, the mechanism of NSAIDs is to act on these cyclooxygenase (COX) enzymes and inhibit them [50, 51].

NSAIDs not only inhibit the production of prostaglandins but also prolong the inflammatory and cartilaginous stage of bone healing by affecting the lineage of chondrocytes, which is written in detail in the following section.

5. Relation of NSAIDs and mature hypertrophied chondrocytes

5.1 Inhibitory effect on differentiation of chondrocytes

The use of NSAIDs in certain patients and *in vitro* studies linked with suppression of chondrocyte proliferation and differentiation [52]. The proliferation and differentiation of chondrocytes and osteoblasts is a critical component of fracture healing from the bone marrow stem cells (BMSCs).

The chondrogenic differentiation in fracture healing undergoes six phases. These phases are mesenchymal cells (chondroprogenitors), condensed mesenchymal cells, chondrocytes, proliferating chondrocytes, pre-hypertrophic chondrocytes, and hypertrophic chondrocytes. The process of chondrogenic differentiation undergoes generalized steps of chondrogenesis, cartilage hypertrophy, and ossification. For the maturation of chondrocytes into mature hypertrophied chondrocytes (MHCs), COX-2 activity is required, but NSAIDs inhibit the formation of MHCs by blocking the COX-2 enzyme (**Figure 5**) [21, 53].

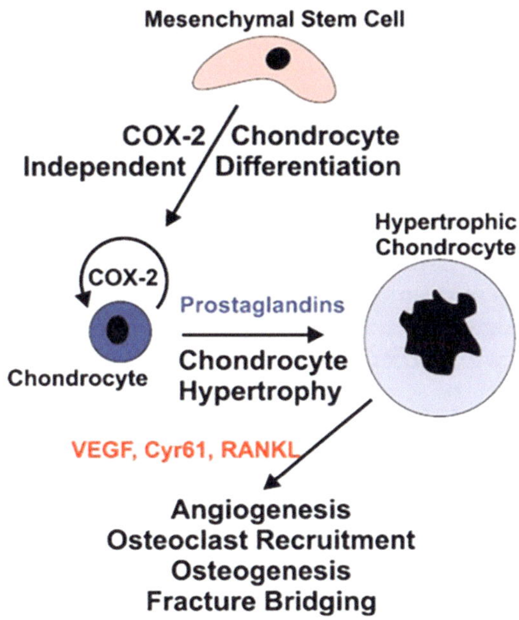

Figure 5.
Role of COX-2 in the formation of hypertrophic chondrocytes [21].

5.2 Negative effect on expression of collagen X

5.2.1 Synthesis, structure, and location of collagen X

Mature Hypertrophied Chondrocytes synthesize collagen X in endochondral ossification. Type X collagen is present within the deep layer of articular cartilage adjacent to the tidemark. Collagen type X is a crucial factor in the successful union of fractures in the tissues going under endochondral ossification [22].

Type X collagen is non-fibrillar collagen consisting of three identical alpha 1 chains, and each chain has three domains: a short triple helix domain flanked by a bigger globular domain at the carboxyl end and a short non-collagenous domain at the amino end [54].

5.2.2 Bone healing marker

COLX is the major marker of hypertrophic chondrocytes, which can be detected within the first few days of bone formation. It plays several important roles contributing to the structural support of the pericellular network that is essential during matrix remodeling and helps in initiating biomineralization [55].

5.2.3 Effects of NSAID

The effects of NSAIDs on collagen type X expression, which is secreted by hypertrophic chondrocytes and an important marker of endochondral ossification during fracture healing, have been investigated in numerous studies. In one previous study, after administration of non-selective NSAIDs (diclofenac sodium and ketorolac) and selective COX-2 NSAIDs, low expression of collagen type X was observed as inhibition of COX enzymes negatively influenced the first phase of chondrogenic differentiation and affect chondrocyte hypertrophy [56]. In another study, a contradicted finding was observed as NSAID treatment did not affect the collagen X expression [57].

6. Relation of NSAIDs and delayed fracture healing

The administration of the NSAIDs during fracture healing can inhibit the formation of PGE2, and the mechanism of action might affect the fracture healing process. Taking into consideration the mechanism of action of NSAIDs, it can be inferred that taking NSAIDs might affect the fracture healing process. However, controversial results were observed when different studies were done on animals and humans.

6.1 Animal studies

Numerous studies have been done in the past in which different results were observed when performed on small animals with the administration of different NSAIDs (**Table 2**) [30].

Year/Study	Model used	Drug	Outcome
Tornkvist et al. [58]	Chicken mesenchymal limb-bud cells	Indomethacin (25–100 μm)	i. No effect on osteogenesis and chondrogenesis
Ho et al. [59]	Osteoblasts derived from fetal rat calvaria	Ketorolac (0.1–1000 μm), Indomethacin (0.01–100 μm)	i. All concentrations of ketorolac inhibited proliferation at 24 hours ii. 0.1 μm of indomethacin or higher inhibited proliferation iii. A dose-dependent increase of Alkaline Phosphate (ALP) was found for concentrations between 0.1 and 100 μm of ketorolac iv. Both NSAIDs stimulated collagen type I synthesis
Evans and Butcher [60]	Human trabecular bone osteoblasts	Indomethacin (0.003–0.3 μm/L)	i. Inhibition of proliferation and increase in collagen synthesis and ALP in a dose-dependent manner
Wang et al. [61]	MG63 human osteoblasts	Celecoxib (1–120 μm)	i. Dose-dependent decrease of cellular proliferation and stimulation of Ca++ production
Chang et al. [62]	Osteoblasts derived from fetal rat calvaria	Diclofenac, piroxicam, indomethacin ketorolac (0.001–0.1 μm)	i. All NSAIDs resulted in cell cycle arrest and cell death ii. Piroxicam had the least effect on producing osteoblastic dysfunction
Wang et al. [63]	Bone Marrow (BM)-derived Rat mesenchymal stem cells	Aspirin 1, 5, 10 mmol/L	i. Inhibition of Mesenchymal stem cells (MSC) proliferation

Year/Study	Model used	Drug	Outcome
Wiontzek et al. [64]	MG63 human osteoblasts	Celecoxib (10 μm)	i. No effect on Ca++ production, COX-2 expression, ALP, and osteocalcin
Wolfesberger et al. [65]	Canine osteosarcoma cell line	Meloxicam (1–200 μg/mL)	i. Marked anti-proliferative effect for concentrations over 100, while lower concentrations resulted in an increase in cell numbers
Chang et al. [66]	Human mesenchymal stem cells and D1-cells (Mice)	Indomethacin (10, 100 μm), celecoxib (1, 10 μm)	i. Inhibition of proliferation for both Nonsteriodal Anti-inflammatory Drugs (NSAIDs) but no significant cytotoxic effect ii. Replenishment of PGE-1, PGE-2 and PGF2a did not reverse this negative effect
Kellinsalmi et al. [67]	Human mesenchymal stem cells	Indomethacin (1, 10, and 100 μm), parecoxib (1, 10, and 100 μm), and NS398 (0.03, 0.3, and 3 μm)	i. All studied NSAIDs-inhibited osteoblastic and osteoclastic differentiation ii. Significant increase of adipocytes suggesting diversion to adipogenesis instead of osteogenesis
Arpornmaeklong et al. [68]	Mouse calvaria cell line MC3T3-E1	Indomethacin (0.1 μm), celecoxib (1.5, 3, and 9 μm)	i. Inhibition of growth with both NSAIDs ii. Indomethacin had a higher inhibitory effect than celecoxib
Abukawa et al. [69]	Porcine BM progenitor cells	Ibuprofen (0.1, 1, 3 mmol/L)	i. 0.1 mmol/L had no effect on proliferation, ALP, or bone matrix mineralization, while inhibition was found for the higher studied concentrations
Chang et al. [70]	Human osteoblasts	Indomethacin (0.1–1 μm), ketorolac (0.1–1 μm), piroxicam (0.1–1 μm), diclofenac (0.1–1 μm), and celecoxib (1–10 μm)	i. Inhibition of proliferation occurred with all studied NSAIDs ii. Replenishment of PGE-1, PGE-2 and PGF2a did not reverse this negative effect
Kolar et al. [71]	MG63 human osteoblasts	Celecoxib (2, 10, and 50 μm)	i. Marginal effect with the concentrations of 2 and 10 μm but 50 μM reduced cell viability and Osteoprotegerin (OPG) secretion and stimulated oxygen consumption and GLUT-1 expression
Yoon et al. [72]	Human bone marrow mesenchymal stem cells	Celecoxib (10, 20, 40 μm), naproxen (100, 200, 300 μm)	i. No effect on ALP and calcium content in the absence of interleukin 1β, while in its presence, ALP and calcium were reduced only with the highest studied concentration

Year/Study	Model used	Drug	Outcome
Guez et al. [73]	Human MG-63 Osteosarcoma cell	Indomethacin (1–10 μm) Nimesulide (1–10 μm) Diclofenac (1–10 μm)	i. All NSAIDs had an inhibiting effect on osteoblastic proliferation and significant effects on the antigenic profile ii. No treatment altered osteocalcin synthesis
Muller et al. [74]	Equine bone marrow mesenchymal stem cells	Flunixin (10–1000 μm), phenylbutazone (10–1000 μm), meloxicam (0.01–200 μm), and celecoxib (0.01–200 μm)	i. Low NSAID concentrations had a positive effect on proliferation, while the higher ones inhibited proliferation ii. Adipogenic and chondrogenic differentiation was found unaltered; however, osteogenesis was significantly disrupted
Pountos et al. [75]	Bone marrow and TB-derived mesenchymal stem cells	Diclofenac, ketorolac, parecoxib, ketoprofen, piroxicam, meloxicam, and lornoxicam (all 0.001 to 100 μg/mL)	i. No effect on MSC proliferation when the cellular medium was supplemented with expected plasma concentrations ii. Negative effect was encountered when high concentrations were used (over 100 μg/mL) iii. NSAIDs in plasma concentrations had no effect on osteogenesis iv. Chondrogenesis was found inhibited by NSAIDs

Table 2.
In vitro studies in animals [30].

6.1.1 Negative effect of NSAIDs

Several animal studies in rodents concluded the negative effect of NSAIDs on fracture repair, bone density, and strength [55]. In an animal experimental study on rat ulna, it was concluded that selective COX-2 inhibitor decreases the area of resorption along the fracture line, and non-selective NSAID administration altered the bone formation and resorption that lead to reduced length decreased remodeling and lamellar bone formation may occur [51]. In another experimental study on rat femur, fracture healing was delayed due to inhibition of COX-2 activity by selective COX-2 inhibitors [76].

Soft callus was seen in the fibula of rabbits due to an increased amount of cartilage and less amount of newly formed bone in callus, indicating delayed fracture healing when treated with non-selective and selective COX-2 inhibitors in a previous study [77]. In another study, it was appreciated that administration of COX-2 inhibitors in rats resulted in delayed healing with poorly developed callus and decreased bone strength [78].

A previous study that examined the effects of non-selective NSAIDs on bone repair in rats concluded that NSAIDs delayed or even completely inhibited fracture healing [79]. Similarly, bone healing was seen delayed with negative effects of systemic inflammation on the repair process in the mice which were given non-selective NSAIDs for 2 weeks after surgery [80].

6.1.2 No effect of NSAIDs

In contrast, in a few other animal studies, there was minor to zero effect on the fracture healing process [70, 71, 81, 82]. NSAIDs-treated groups showed no significant effect on fracture healing and remodeling in the animals [81]. The administration of NSAIDs did not affect fracture healing when given to rats after closed diaphyseal fibula fractures [73].

6.2 Human studies

Numerous previous studies have been done in humans, with the administration of different NSAIDs for certain time durations, and different results have been obtained (**Table 3**).

6.2.1 Negative effect of NSAIDs

In human studies, the administration of NSAIDs also resulted in controversial effects on the fracture healing process. In one human study, it was concluded that prolonged high-dose exposure to NSAIDs inhibits osteogenesis, leading to malunion and non-union in adults [74].

In another human retrospective study, malunion and non-union were seen in patients treated with both non-selective and selective COX-2 NSAIDs administration for more than 1 week, whereas delayed bone healing was seen in patients who had taken NSAIDs for 1 week, confirming the relationship between the duration of the treatment and fracture healing process [93].

6.2.2 No effect of NSAIDs

There are also a few studies that concluded NSAIDs have no effect on the fracture healing process. As in one previous study, no effect on fracture healing was seen between patients of Colles fracture who had been treated with ibuprofen and placebo for 2 week [94].

7. Conclusion

The conclusion drawn from the preceding discussion underscores the critical impact of non-steroidal anti-inflammatory drugs (NSAIDs), both non-selective and selective COX-2 inhibitors, on the process of fracture healing. Through their mechanism of action, these medications have been shown to detrimentally affect the expression of collagen X during the initial phases of fracture healing. This downregulation of collagen X expression is strongly associated with decreased new bone formation, leading to an increased presence of bone defects and fibrous tissue at the fracture site. As such, NSAIDs, particularly non-selective COX inhibitors, pose a significant risk to the optimal progression of bone healing.

Year/Study	Design	Drug	Conclusions and recommendations
Davis and Ackroyd [83]	Prospective double-blinded study of 100 patients with Colles' fracture	Flurbiprofen (50 mg TDS)	i. No effect on Colles' fracture
Adolphson et al. [84]	Randomized double-blinded study on 42 postmenopausal women with Colles fracture	Piroxicam	i. No decrease in the rate of fracture healing ii. Patients receiving piroxicam had iii. significantly less pain iv. No difference in the rate of functional v. Recovery
Butcher and Marsh [85]	Retrospective review of 94 patients with tibial fracture	Not specified	i. Increase in the length of time to the union by 7.6 weeks ($P = 0.0003$) (16.7 weeks versus 24.3 weeks)
Wurnig et al. [86]	80 prospective patients receiving indomethacin prophylaxis for THR compared with 82 patients without	Indomethacin (oral 50 mg BD)	i. No effect on prosthetic loosening after cementless hip arthroplasty
Giannoudis et al. [87]	Retrospective review of 377 patients treated with IM nail	Ibuprofen and diclofenac	i. Increased risk for non-union in patients receiving NSAIDs
Bhandari et al. [88]	Retrospective review of 192 tibial shaft fractures	Not specified	i. Relative risk of 2.02 ($P = 0.035$) for patients who take NSAIDs
Burd et al. [89]	Retrospective review of 282 with acetabular fractures	Indomethacin	i. Patients receiving indomethacin had an increased risk of developing non-union
Sculean et al. [90]	Randomized blinded study on 20 patients with deep intra-bony defect	Rofecoxib (25 mg/day for 14 days)	i. No effect on the healing of intra-bony periodontal defects
Bhattacharyya et al. [91]	Retrospective review of 9995 humeral shaft fractures treated non-operatively	Not specified	i. Exposure to non-selective NSAIDs in the period 61–90 days after a humeral shaft fracture was associated with non-union
Meunier et al. [92]	Randomized study involving 50 patients undergoing total knee replacement	Celecoxib (200 mg BD)	i. No differences in prosthesis migration, pain scores, range of motion, and subjective outcome were found after 2 years

Table 3.
Studies analyzing the effect of NSAIDs on bone healing in humans [30].

The implications of this finding are profound, especially in clinical settings where fracture healing is of paramount importance. Patients who are administered NSAIDs, especially non-selective COX inhibitors, may experience delayed healing processes, prolonged recovery times, and increased susceptibility to complications associated with inadequate bone regeneration. It is imperative, therefore, for healthcare providers to exercise caution when prescribing NSAIDs, particularly in individuals deemed to be at considerable risk for impaired bone healing.

Furthermore, this conclusion underscores the need for a nuanced approach to pain management in patients with fractures, particularly in those who are vulnerable to compromised bone healing. While NSAIDs are often prescribed for their analgesic and anti-inflammatory properties, their potential adverse effects on bone metabolism and healing cannot be overlooked. Healthcare providers must weigh the benefits of pain relief against the potential risks of impaired fracture healing when making treatment decisions for their patients.

Considering these findings, it is recommended that alternative pain management strategies be considered for patients at risk of impaired bone healing. This may include the use of alternative analgesic medications or adjunctive therapies that do not interfere with the process of bone regeneration.

Additionally, close monitoring of patients who require NSAID therapy for other medical conditions is essential to promptly detect any signs of delayed fracture healing. Moving forward, further research is warranted to elucidate the precise mechanisms by which NSAIDs modulate fracture healing and to identify potential strategies to mitigate their adverse effects. A better understanding of these mechanisms will enable healthcare providers to optimize pain management strategies while minimizing the risk of impaired bone healing in vulnerable patient populations.

In the end, the use of non-selective and selective COX-2 NSAIDs has been shown to negatively impact fracture healing by decreasing the expression of collagen X and impairing new bone formation. Healthcare providers must exercise caution when prescribing NSAIDs, particularly in patients at risk of impaired bone healing. Alternative pain management strategies should be considered, and close monitoring of patients receiving NSAID therapy is essential to ensure optimal outcomes in fracture healing. Further research is needed to elucidate the underlying mechanisms and develop targeted interventions to mitigate the adverse effects of NSAIDs on bone healing.

Author details

Rana Muhammad Zeeshan
Islam Medical College, Sialkot, Pakistan

*Address all correspondence to: shani3687@gmail.com

References

[1] McVeigh LG et al. Assessment, quantification, and Management of Fracture Pain: From animals to the clinic. Current Osteoporosis Reports. 2020;**18**(5):460-470. DOI: 10.1007/s11914-020-00617-z

[2] Murphy PB et al. Efficacy and safety of non-steroidal anti-inflammatory drugs (NSAIDs) for the treatment of acute pain after orthopedic trauma: A practice management guideline from the eastern Association for the Surgery of trauma and the orthopedic trauma association. Trauma Surgery & Acute Care Open. 2023;**8**(1):e001056. DOI: 10.1136/tsaco-2022-001056

[3] Peng J et al. Bulleyaconitine a reduces fracture-induced pain and promotes fracture healing in mice. Frontiers in Pharmacology. 2023;**14**:1046514. DOI: 10.3389/fphar.2023.1046514

[4] Wibowo H, Widiyanti P. The effect of diclofenac sodium on callus formation in white male rat (Rattus norvegicus) cruris fracture healing. Journal of Folia Medica Indonesiana. 2022;**58**(2):108-112. DOI: 10.20473/fmi.v58i2.25212

[5] Wu A-M et al. Global, regional, and national burden of bone fractures in 204 countries and territories, 1990-2019: A systematic analysis from the global burden of disease study 2019. The Lancet. 2021;**2**(9):e580-e592. DOI: 10.1016/S2666-7568(21)00172-0

[6] Zhao Y et al. Chronic pain after bone fracture: Current insights into molecular mechanisms and therapeutic strategies. Brain Sciences. 2022;**12**(8):1056. DOI: 10.3390/brainsci12081056

[7] Shenoy R, Pillai A. Biology of fracture healing-an overview. Journal of Thoracic Oncology. 2017;**05**(2):283-293. Available from: www.researchgate.net/publication/318573942_Biology_of_fracture_healing__an_overview

[8] Kostenuik P, Mirza FM. Fracture healing physiology and the quest for therapies for delayed healing and nonunion. Journal of Orthopaedic Research. 2017;**35**(2):213-223. DOI: 10.1002/jor.23460

[9] Bigham-Sadegh A, Oryan A. Basic concepts regarding fracture healing and the current options and future directions in managing bone fractures. International Wound Journal. 2015;**12**(3):238-247. DOI: 10.1111/iwj.12231

[10] Ghiasi MS et al. Bone fracture healing in mechanobiological modeling: A review of principles and methods. Bone Reports. 2017;**6**:87-100. DOI: 10.1016/j.bonr.2017.03.002

[11] Marsell R, Einhorn TA. The biology of fracture healing. Injury. 2011;**42**(6):551-555. DOI: 10.1016/j.injury.2011.03.031

[12] Ghimire S et al. The investigation of bone fracture healing under intramembranous and endochondral ossification. Bone Reports. 2021;**14**:100740. DOI: 10.1016/j.bonr.2020.100740

[13] Wang W, Yeung KWK. Bone grafts and biomaterials substitutes for bone defect repair: A review. Bioactive Materials. 2017;**2**(4):224-247. DOI: 10.1016/j.bioactmat.2017.05.007

[14] Bahney CS et al. Cellular biology of fracture healing. Journal of Orthopaedic Research. 2019;**37**(1):35-50. DOI: 10.1002/jor.24170

[15] Auer JA, Stick JA. Equine Surgery-E-Book. Elsevier Health Sciences; 2018. DOI: 10.1111/j.1751-0813.2012.00923.x. Available from: https://www.academia.edu/43994994/Equine_Surgery

[16] Kolar P et al. The early fracture hematoma and its potential role in fracture healing. Tissue Engineering Part B: Reviews. 2010;**16**(4):427-434. DOI: 10.1089/ten.TEB.2009.0687

[17] Ho-Shui-Ling A et al. Bone regeneration strategies: Engineered scaffolds, bioactive molecules and stem cells current stage and future perspectives. Biomaterials. 2018;**180**:143-162. DOI: 10.1016/j.biomaterials.2018.07.017

[18] Oryan A, Monazzah S, Bigham-Sadegh A. Bone injury and fracture healing biology. Biomedical and Environmental Sciences. 2015;**28**(1):57-71. DOI: 10.3967/bes2015.006

[19] Schindeler A et al. Bone remodeling during fracture repair: The cellular picture. Seminars in Cell & Developmental Biology. 2008;**19**(5):459-466. DOI: 10.1016/j.semcdb.2008.07.004

[20] Bahrambeigi S et al. Metformin; an old antidiabetic drug with new potentials in bone disorders. Biomedical and Pharmacology Journal. 2019;**109**:1593-1601. DOI: 10.1016/j.biopha.2018.11.032

[21] Su B, O'Connor JP. NSAID therapy effects on healing of bone, tendon, and the enthesis. Journal of Applied Physiology. 2013;**115**(6):892-899. DOI: 10.1152/japplphysiol.00053.2013

[22] Topping RE, Bolander ME, Balian G. Type X collagen in fracture callus and the effects of experimental diabetes. Clinical Orthopaedics and Related Research. 1994;**308**:220-228. DOI: 10.1097/00003086-199411000-00032

[23] Yang L et al. Hypertrophic chondrocytes can become osteoblasts and osteocytes in endochondral bone formation. Proceedings of the National Academy of Sciences. 2014;**111**(33):12097-12102. DOI: 10.1073/pnas.1302703111

[24] Runyan CM, Gabrick KS. Biology of bone formation, fracture healing, and distraction osteogenesis. The Journal of Craniofacial Surgery. 2017;**28**(5):1380-1389. DOI: 10.1097/SCS.0000000000003625

[25] Baht GS, Vi L, Alman BA. The role of the immune cells in fracture healing. Current Osteoporosis Reports. 2018;**16**(2):138-145. DOI: 10.1007/s11914-018-0423-2

[26] Poniatowski Ł, A., et al., Transforming growth factor beta family: Insight into the role of growth factors in regulation of fracture healing biology and potential clinical applications. Mediators of Inflammation, 2015. 2015: p. 137823. DOI: 10.1155/2015/137823

[27] Dekel S, Lenthall G, Francis M. Release of prostaglandins from bone and muscle after tibial fracture. An experimental study in rabbits. Journal of Bone and Joint Surgery. 1981;**63**(2):185-189. DOI: 10.1302/0301-620X.63B2.7217139

[28] Hatakeyama Y, Tuan RS, Shum L. Distinct functions of BMP4 and GDF5 in the regulation of chondrogenesis. Journal of Cellular Biochemistry. 2004;**91**(6):1204-1217. DOI: 10.1002/jcb.20019

[29] O'Connor JP et al. Fracture healing and lipid mediators. Bonekey Reports. 2014;**3**:517. DOI: 10.1038/bonekey.2014.12

[30] Pountos I et al. Do nonsteroidal anti-inflammatory drugs affect bone

healing? A critical analysis. Scientific World Journal. 2012;**2012**:606404. DOI: 10.1100/2012/606404

[31] Mayes PA, Botham KM. Lipids of physiologic significance 14. In: Harper's Illustrated Biochemistry. Lange; 2003. p. 111. Available from: https://www.academia.edu/41472638/Harpers_Illustrated_Biochemistry_a_LANGE_medical_book_twenty_sixth_edition_Medical_Publishing_Division

[32] Ricciotti E, FitzGerald GA. Prostaglandins and inflammation. Arteriosclerosis, Thrombosis, and Vascular Biology. 2011;**31**(5):986-1000. DOI: 10.1161/ATVBAHA.110.207449

[33] Graham S et al. Prostaglandin EP2 and EP4 receptor agonists in bone formation and bone healing: *In vivo* and *in vitro* evidence. Expert Opinion on Investigational Drugs. 2009;**18**(6):749-766. DOI: 10.1517/13543780902893051

[34] Hubich A, Sholukh MJB. Biochemistry of prostaglandins A. Biochemistry (Mosc.). 2006;**71**(3):229-238. DOI: 10.1134/s0006297906030011

[35] Funk CD. Prostaglandins and leukotrienes: Advances in eicosanoid biology. Science. 2001;**294**(5548):1871-1875. DOI: 10.1126/science.294.5548.1871

[36] Rouzer CA, Marnett LJ. Cyclooxygenases: Structural and functional insights. Journal of Lipid Research. 2009;**50 Suppl**(Suppl):S29-S34. DOI: 10.1194/jlr.R800042-JLR200

[37] Sales KJ, Jabbour HN. Cyclooxygenase enzymes and prostaglandins in pathology of the endometrium. Reproduction. 2003;**126**(5):559-567. DOI: 10.1530/rep.0.1260559

[38] Li M, Thompson DD, Paralkar VM. Prostaglandin E(2) receptors in bone formation. International Orthopaedics. 2007;**31**(6):767-772. DOI: 10.1007/s00264-007-0406-x

[39] Fracon RN et al. Prostaglandins and bone: Potential risks and benefits related to the use of nonsteroidal anti-inflammatory drugs in clinical dentistry. Journal of Oral Science. 2008;**50**(3):247-252. DOI: 10.2334/josnusd.50.247

[40] Geusens P et al. NSAIDs and fracture healing. Current Opinion in Rheumatology. 2013;**25**(4):524-531. DOI: 10.1097/BOR.0b013e32836200b8

[41] Bacchi S et al. Clinical pharmacology of non-steroidal anti-inflammatory drugs: A review. Anti-Inflammatory & Anti-Allergy Agents in Medicinal Chemistry. 2012;**11**(1):52-64. DOI: 10.2174/187152312803476255

[42] Chen L. Current trends in PGE2 targeting for anti-inflammatory therapy. Pharmaceutical Bioprocessing. 2016;**4**(3):52-53. Available from: https://www.openaccessjournals.com/articles/current-trends-in-pge2-targeting-for-antiinflammatory-therapy.html

[43] Wheeler P, Batt ME. Do non-steroidal anti-inflammatory drugs adversely affect stress fracture healing? A short review. British Journal of Sports Medicine. 2005;**39**(2):65-69. DOI: 10.1136/bjsm.2004.012492

[44] Burian M, Geisslinger G. COX-dependent mechanisms involved in the antinociceptive action of NSAIDs at central and peripheral sites. Pharmacology & Therapeutics. 2005;**107**(2):139-154. DOI: 10.1016/j.pharmthera.2005.02.004

[45] Tomić M et al. Chapter 1 - clinical uses of nonsteroidal anti-inflammatory drugs (NSAIDs) and potential benefits of NSAIDs modified-release preparations.

In: Čalija B, editor. Microsized and Nanosized Carriers for Nonsteroidal Anti-Inflammatory Drugs. Boston: Academic Press; 2017. pp. 1-29. DOI: 10.1016/B978-0-12-804017-1.00001-7

[46] Rao CV, Reddy BS. NSAIDs and chemoprevention. Current Cancer Drug Targets. 2004;**4**(1):29-42. DOI: 10.2174/1568009043481632

[47] Ghlichloo I, Gerriets V. Nonsteroidal Anti-Inflammatory Drugs (NSAIDs). Treasure Island (FL): StatPearls Publishing LLC; 2022. Available from: https://www.ncbi.nlm.nih.gov/books/NBK547742/

[48] Prior C, Eisen D, Herlands L. Use of NSAIDs for Prevention and Treatment of Cellular Abnormalities of the Female Reproductive Tract. World Intellectual Property Organization. Google Patents; 2003, Available from: https://patents.google.com/patent/US20030004143A1/en; https://patentscope.wipo.int/search/docs2/pct/WO2002085327/pdf/Mbg6jVcvLeByL7V3VzkmedZKlh89dRevNCf6f7TWv38

[49] Ishiguro H, Kawahara T. Nonsteroidal anti-inflammatory drugs and prostatic diseases. BioMed Research International. 2014;**2014**:436123. DOI: 10.1155/2014/436123

[50] Gunaydin C, Bilge SS. Effects of nonsteroidal anti-inflammatory drugs at the molecular level. The Eurasian Journal of Medicine. 2018;**50**(2):116-121. DOI: 10.5152/eurasianjmed.2018.0010

[51] Kidd LJ et al. Selective and non-selective cyclooxygenase inhibitors delay stress fracture healing in the rat ulna. Journal of Orthopaedic Research. 2013;**31**(2):235-242. DOI: 10.1002/jor.22203

[52] Karaarslan N et al. Effect of naproxen on proliferation and differentiation of primary cell cultures isolated from human cartilage tissue. Experimental and Therapeutic Medicine. 2018;**16**(3):1647-1654. DOI: 10.3892/etm.2018.6351

[53] Jin F et al. The role of chondrocytes in fracture healing. Journal of Spine. 2016;**5**(4):1-8. DOI: 10.4172/2165-7939.1000328

[54] He Y et al. Type X collagen levels are elevated in serum from human osteoarthritis patients and associated with biomarkers of cartilage degradation and inflammation. BMC Musculoskeletal Disorders. 2014;**15**(1):1-10. DOI: 10.1186/1471-2474-15-309

[55] Knuth C et al. Collagen type X is essential for successful mesenchymal stem cell-mediated cartilage formation and subsequent endochondral ossification. European Journal of Cell Biology. 2019;**38**:106-122. DOI: 10.22203/eCM.v038a09

[56] Merkely G et al. Do nonsteroidal anti-inflammatory drugs have a deleterious effect on cartilage repair? A systematic review. Cartilage. 2021;**13**(1_suppl):326s-341s. DOI: 10.1177/1947603519855770

[57] Kalaszczynska I, Ferdyn K. Wharton's jelly derived mesenchymal stem cells: Future of regenerative medicine? Recent findings and clinical significance. BioMed Research International. 2015;**2015**:430847. DOI: 10.1155/2015/430847

[58] Tornkvist B et al. Lack of effect of indomethacin on mesenchymal limb-bud cells in vitro. Acta Orthopaedica Scandinavica. 1984;**55**(3):378-380. DOI: 10.3109/17453678408992379

[59] Ho ML et al. Effects of nonsteroidal anti-inflammatory drugs and prostaglandins on osteoblastic

functions. Biochemical Pharmacology. 1999;**58**(6):983-990. DOI: 10.1016/s0006-2952(99)00186-0

[60] Evans CE, Butcher C. The influence on human osteoblasts in vitro of non-steroidal anti-inflammatory drugs which act on different cyclooxygenase enzymes. The Journal of Bone and Joint Surgery. British Volume. 2004;**86**(3):444-449. DOI: 10.1302/0301-620X.86B3.14592

[61] Wang JL et al. Effect of celecoxib on Ca2+ movement and cell proliferation in human osteoblasts. Biochemical Pharmacology. 2004;**67**(6):1123-1130. DOI: 10.1016/j.bcp.2003.11.004

[62] Chang JK et al. Nonsteroidal anti-inflammatory drug effects on osteoblastic cell cycle, cytotoxicity, and cell death. Connective Tissue Research. 2005;**46**(4-5):200-210. DOI: 10.1080/03008200500344025

[63] Wang Y et al. Growth inhibition of mesenchymal stem cells by aspirin: Involvement of the WNT/beta-catenin signal pathway. Clinical and Experimental Pharmacology and Physiology. 2006;**33**(8):696-701. DOI: 10.1111/j.1440-1681.2006.04432.x

[64] Wiontzek M et al. Effects of dexamethasone and celecoxib on calcium homeostasis and expression of cyclooxygenase-2 mRNA in MG-63 human osteosarcoma cells. Clinical and Experimental Rheumatology. 2006;**24**(4):366-372. Available from: https://www.clinexprheumatol.org/article.asp?a=2889

[65] Wolfesberger B et al. In vitro effects of meloxicam with or without doxorubicin on canine osteosarcoma cells. Journal of Veterinary Pharmacology and Therapeutics. 2006;**29**(1):15-23. DOI: 10.1111/j.1365-2885.2006.00704.x

[66] Chang JK et al. Effects of anti-inflammatory drugs on proliferation, cytotoxicity and osteogenesis in bone marrow mesenchymal stem cells. Biochemical Pharmacology. 2007;**74**(9):1371-1382. DOI: 10.1016/j.bcp.2007.06.047

[67] Kellinsalmi M et al. Inhibition of cyclooxygenase-2 down-regulates osteoclast and osteoblast differentiation and favours adipocyte formation in vitro. European Journal of Pharmacology. 2007;**572**(2-3):102-110. DOI: 10.1016/j.ejphar.2007.06.030

[68] Arpornmaeklong P, Akarawatcharangura B, Pripatnanont P. Factors influencing effects of specific COX-2 inhibitor NSAIDs on growth and differentiation of mouse osteoblasts on titanium surfaces. The International Journal of Oral & Maxillofacial Implants. 2008;**23**(6):1071-1081. Available from: http://medlib.yu.ac.kr/eur_j_oph/ijom/IJOMI/ijomi_23_1071.pdf

[69] Abukawa H et al. Effect of ibuprofen on osteoblast differentiation of porcine bone marrow-derived progenitor cells. Journal of Oral and Maxillofacial Surgery. 2009;**67**(11):2412-2417. DOI: 10.1016/j.joms.2009.05.434

[70] Hak DJ et al. The effect of cox-2 specific inhibition on direct fracture healing in the rabbit tibia. Journal of Orthopaedic Science. 2011;**16**(1):93-98. DOI: 10.1007/s00776-010-0016-0

[71] Karachalios T et al. The effects of the short-term administration of low therapeutic doses of anti-COX-2 agents on the healing of fractures: An experimental study in rabbits. Journal of Bone and Joint Surgery. 2007;**89**(9):1253-1260. DOI: 10.1302/0301-620X.89B9.19050

[72] Al-Waeli H et al. Non-steroidal anti-inflammatory drugs and bone

healing in animal models-a systematic review and meta-analysis. Systematic Reviews. 2021;**10**(1):201. DOI: 10.1186/s13643-021-01690-w

[73] Inal S et al. Comparison of the effects of dexketoprofen trometamol, meloxicam and diclofenac sodium on fibular fracture healing, kidney and liver: An experimental rat model. Injury. 2014;**45**(3):494-500. DOI: 10.1016/j.injury.2013.10.002

[74] Wheatley BM et al. Effect of NSAIDs on bone healing rates: A meta-analysis. The Journal of the American Academy of Orthopaedic Surgeons. 2019;**27**(7):e330-e336. DOI: 10.5435/JAAOS-D-17-00727

[75] Pountos I et al. NSAIDS inhibit in vitro MSC chondrogenesis but not osteogenesis: Implications for mechanism of bone formation inhibition in man. Journal of Cellular and Molecular Medicine. 2011;**15**(3):525-534. DOI: 10.1111/j.1582-4934.2010.01006.x

[76] Simon AM, Manigrasso MB, O'Connor JP. Cyclo-oxygenase 2 function is essential for bone fracture healing. Journal of Bone and Mineral Research. 2002;**17**(6):963-976. DOI: 10.1359/jbmr.2002.17.6.963

[77] O'Connor JP et al. A comparison of the effects of ibuprofen and rofecoxib on rabbit fibula osteotomy healing. Acta Orthopaedica. 2009;**80**(5):597-605. DOI: 10.3109/17453670903316769

[78] Herbenick MA et al. Effects of a cyclooxygenase 2 inhibitor on fracture healing in a rat model. The American Journal of Orthopedics. 2008;**37**(7):E133-E137. Available from: https://cdn.mdedge.com/files/s3fs-public/Document/September-2017/037070133e.pdf

[79] Lu LY et al. Pro-inflammatory M1 macrophages promote osteogenesis by mesenchymal stem cells via the COX-2-prostaglandin E2 pathway. Journal of Orthopaedic Research. 2017;**35**(11):2378-2385. DOI: 10.1002/jor.23553

[80] Ramirez-Garcia-Luna JL et al. Defective bone repair in diclofenac treated C57Bl6 mice with and without lipopolysaccharide induced systemic inflammation. Journal of Cellular Physiology. 2019;**234**(3):3078-3087. DOI: 10.1002/jcp.27128

[81] Brown KM et al. Effect of COX-2-specific inhibition on fracture-healing in the rat femur. Journal of Bone and Joint Surgery. 2004;**86**(1):116-123. DOI: 10.2106/00004623-200401000-00017

[82] Goodman SB et al. Temporal effects of a COX-2-selective NSAID on bone ingrowth. Journal of Biomedical Materials Research Part A. 2005;**72**(3):279-287. DOI: 10.1002/jbm.a.30231

[83] Davis TR, Ackroyd CE. Non-steroidal anti-inflammatory agents in the management of Colles' fractures. British Journal of Clinical Pharmacology. 1988;**42**(5):184-189. DOI: 10.1111/j.1742-1241.1988.tb08548.x

[84] Adolphson P et al. No effects of piroxicam on osteopenia and recovery after Colles' fracture. A randomized, double-blind, placebo-controlled, prospective trial. Archives of Orthopaedic and Trauma Surgery. 1993;**112**(3):127-130. DOI: 10.1007/bf00449987

[85] Butcher C, Marsh DJI. Nonsteroidal anti-inflammatory drugs delay tibial fracture union. 1996;**27**:375. Available from: https://www.infona.pl//resource/bwmeta1.element.elsevier-9a95db63-612e-3703-9857-b00439a481d3

[86] Wurnig C et al. Six-year results of a cementless stem with prophylaxis against heterotopic bone. Clinical Orthopaedics and Related Research. 1999;**8**:150-158. DOI: 10.1097/00003086-199904000-00020

[87] Giannoudis PV et al. Nonunion of the femoral diaphysis. The influence of reaming and nonsteroidal anti-inflammatory drugs. The Journal of Bone and Joint Surgery. 2000;**82**:655-658. DOI: 10.1302/0301-620x.82b5.9899

[88] Bhandari M et al. Predictors of reoperation following operative management of fractures of the tibial shaft. Journal of Orthopaedic Trauma. 2003;**17**:353-361. DOI: 10.1097/00005131-200305000-00006

[89] Burd TA et al. Heterotopic ossification prophylaxis with indomethacin increases the risk of long-bone nonunion. The Journal of Bone and Joint Surgery. 2003;**85**:700-705. DOI: 10.1302/0301-620X.85B5.13970

[90] Sculean A et al. The effect of postsurgical administration of a selective cyclo-oxygenase-2 inhibitor on the healing of intrabony defects following treatment with enamel matrix proteins. Clinical Oral Investigations. 2003;**7**:108-112. DOI: 10.1007/s00784-003-0200-0

[91] Bhattacharyya T et al. Nonsteroidal anti-inflammatory drugs and nonunion of humeral shaft fractures. Arthritis & Rheumatology. 2005;**53**:364-367. DOI: 10.1002/art.21170

[92] Meunier A et al. Celecoxib does not appear to affect prosthesis fixation in total knee replacement: A randomized study using radiostereometry in 50 patients. Acta Orthopaedica. 2009;**80**:46-50. DOI: 10.1080/17453670902804976

[93] Lisowska B, Kosson D, Domaracka K. Positives and negatives of nonsteroidal anti-inflammatory drugs in bone healing: The effects of these drugs on bone repair. Drug Design, Development and Therapy. 2018;**12**:1809-1814. DOI: 10.2147/DDDT.S164565

[94] Aliuskevicius M, Østgaard SE, Rasmussen S. No influence of ibuprofen on bone healing after Colles' fracture - a randomized controlled clinical trial. Injury. 2019;**50**(7):1309-1317. DOI: 10.1002/jor.24498

Chapter 3

Bone Development and Growth

Ayesha Bashir, Qurrat ul Ain, Naveeda Bashir and Wajahat Sohail

Abstract

Osteogenesis is a complex process of bone formation involving several phases and utilizes various cell, metabolites, hormones, and organic and inorganics components. Numerous genetic factors mediate bone formation. Initially, progenitor cells produce osteoblastic lines, which pass through three major cell differentiation stages: proliferation, maturation of matrix, and mineralization. Based on embryonic origin, ossification is of two types: intramembranous and endochondral. In intramembranous ossification, mesenchymal cells in ossification center directly differentiate into osteoblasts, without prior cartilage formation. It involves mesenchymal cell proliferation in highly vascularized areas of embryonic connective tissue, leading to primary ossification center formation. These cells then synthesize bone matrix at periphery, with continuous differentiation into osteoblasts. The resulting bone undergoes reshaping and is eventually replaced by mature lamellar bone. Sufficient blood supply and communication among cells by lacunar-canalicular system are crucial for bone synthesis and maintenance. In contrast, endochondral ossification begins with the formation of primary ossification center within cartilage. Chondrocytes undergo proliferation, expanding the cartilage through cartilage matrix deposition. Central region of cartilage sees the maturation of chondrocytes into hypertrophic chondrocytes. As primary ossification center forms, marrow cavity expands toward epiphysis. The process is completed by subsequent stages of endochondral ossification in various zones of ossification.

Keywords: osteogenesis, remodeling, RANK/RANKL/OPG signaling, ossification, osteocytes, osteoblasts, osteoclasts

1. Introduction

Bone is the toughest connective tissue in the human body, consisting of 50% water and other solid elements that involve several minerals. Specifically, 33% of cellular material is made up of 76% calcium salt. The bone's primary source of nutrition throughout development is the blood supply, and hormones play a fundamental role in regulating this process. Osteoblasts, osteoclasts, and other bone-forming cells are responsible for determining new bone growth [1].

Bone serves three major purpose: firstly, it plays a crucial role in maintaining calcium homeostasis and works as a storehouse of phosphate (PO_4^{3-}), potassium

(K^+), magnesium (Mg^+), and bicarbonate ($H1CO_3^-$). Secondly, it provides protection to internal organs and mechanical support to soft tissues and acts as a lever for muscle contraction. This supports bodily functions, including mobility. And lastly, it is the primary site of hematopoiesis in adults [2].

The bone matrix is different from matrices of other connective tissue in regards that it regenerates continuously throughout the life because of bone turnover and physiological mineralization. Bone tissue has mineral as well as non-mineral constituents. On (and inside) the bone tissue, there are three different types of cells: (a) the osteoblasts that build new bone, which transform into (b) osteocytes when osteoblasts absorb mineral and (c) the osteoclasts that destroy or break down new bone. These cells communicate and interact with each another through signaling substance or direct cell contact [3].

1.1 Bone cells

The primary functions of bone cells, originating from the mesenchymal stem (MSCs) and hematopoietic stem cell (HSCs) lines, are the absorption of bone and remodeling of bone. Bone cells are divided into many categories according to their appearance, function, and distinct location [4]. A mature osteoblast has an enormous quantity of RER and huge Golgi apparatus. Some of the osteoblasts possess cytoplasmic projections in order to travel in bone matrix direction and finally reached at osteocyte process. At this stage, this OB has two choices: either they convert into osteocyte or BLCs or undergo programmed cell death. Surprisingly in the vacuoles of osteoblasts, there are some ovoid bodies having dense bodies, and some TUNEL-positive structures are found and seen. These findings indicate that they are also able to engulf apoptotic materials in addition to skilled phagocytosis during the alveolar development of bone (**Figure 1**) [2].

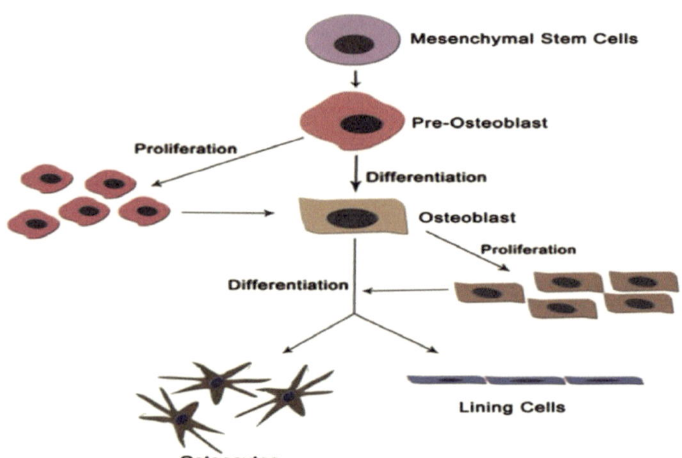

Figure 1.
Classification of bone cells as osteoblasts, osteoclast bone-lining cells, and osteocytes on the basis of their source, resorption, development, and functions. Mature osteoblast structure as a single cuboidal cell layer having enormous quantity of RER and huge Golgi apparatus.

1.2 Osteoblasts

The main cells responsible for forming bones are known as osteoblasts (OBs). These cells are in cuboidal and plump-like appearance and are organized in different layers to form matrix which is then mineralized extracellularly. Osteoblasts comes from mesenchymal stem cells (MSCs) that produce tendon fibroblasts, fat, muscle, or chondrocytes, as well as other types of fibroblasts [5].

For MSCs, to commit osteo-progenitor lineage, several genes must be expressed. This includes components of Wnt pathway and bone morphogenetic protein (BMP) synthesis. Osteoblast differentiation is basically based on expressions and activation of RUNX2, osteorix (Osx), and Dlx5. Among them, RUNX is considered more important for their differentiation because it upregulates CollA1, BSP, and BGLAP as well as ALP and OCN (**Figure 2**).

After the expression of CollA1 and RUNX2, there starts a proliferation phase. At this stage, precursors of osteoblasts are referred to as pre-osteoblasts because they show alkaline phosphatase (ALP) activity.

Some transitions indicate the conversion of pre-osteoblast to mature OBs. This includes elevation of Osx synthesis and release of some bone matrix proteins. Additionally, configuration of osteoblasts changes, converting into large cuboidal-cells.

Other elements such as connexin 43, microRNAs, and fibroblast growth factor (FGF) are crucial for the differentiation of osteoblasts.

After the matrix formation, a new phase starts having two sub-stages, that is, vesicular and fibrillary stage in which matrix mineralization occurs. Organic matrix deposition and their mineralization are the two major steps for bone matrix formation through osteoblasts. During the initial stage, bone matrix is formed by the release of collagen type 1, non-collagenous proteins such as OCN, osteopontin, and BSPII, and proteoglycans such as biglycan or decorin.

After the matrix formation, a new phase starts having two sub-stages, that is, vesicular and fibrillary stage in which matrix mineralization occurs. Matrix vesicle

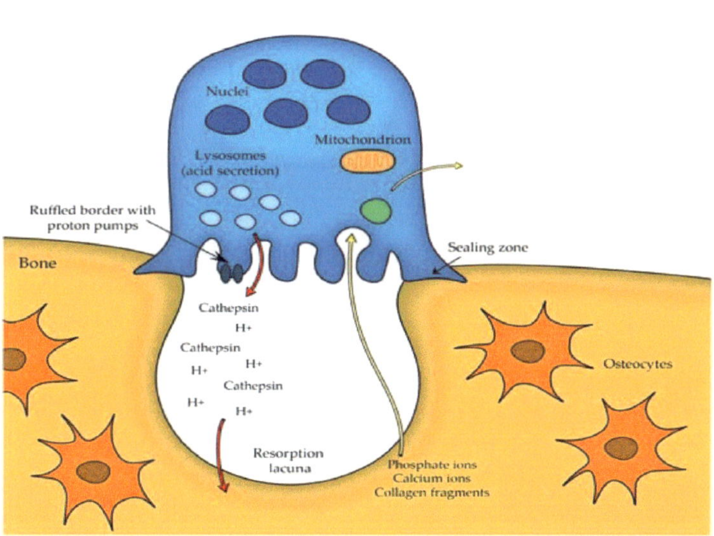

Figure 2.
Osteoblast transformation after the bone-forming phase, the sealing zone, and ruffle border and ionic transport.

releases from domains of membrane and connects to other substances as well as proteoglycans (PGs) in the vesicular phase. Ca^{2+} immobilizes these PGs. These Ca^{2+} release through some channels which are created by annexin protein when there is disintegration of PGs [6].

1.3 Bone lining cells

In contrast to osteoblasts that are present on the bone surface, these are some flat or thin barely noticeable cells which surrounds the bony inactive surface of the human skeleton. Initially, bone lining cells (BLCs) were considered to be preosteoblasts. Currently, it is accepted that osteoblasts that fail to suffer apoptosis and fail to differentiate into osteocytes become bone lining cells [7].

Although BLCs are present on many bone surfaces, but they are well-characterized on endosteal and endocortical surfaces. The majority of the skeletal surface is covered with BLCs and is inactive. Only a small percentage of the overall skeletal surface is remodeling at any one moment. Whereas, BLCs cover the non-remodeling or "inactive" bone surfaces. It is likely that these surfaces, together with the cells connected to them, are physiologically functioning in terms of mineral balance and calcium exchange. BLCs are flattened across the outside of the bone such that they seem exceedingly thin and elongated when sliced perpendicular to the surface. By light microscopy, it can be hard to differentiate BLCs from diverse cell types, including adventitial, stromal, marrow sac, and osteoprogenitor cells. Through gap junctions, they establish connections with neighboring bone lining cells (BLCs) and send cell processes into surface canaliculi.

Another ability that BLCs have is that they can differentiate into osteogenic cells; that is why, they act as a determined osteogenic precursor's source. Along with other endosteal tissue cells, BLCs may do some crucial job in hematopoiesis and may be a key element of the marrow stromal system, possibly by regulating the inductive microenvironment. BLCs may play a role in the initiation of bone resorption and remodeling by transmitting the activation signal. Also, evidence illustrates the importance of BLCs in maintaining bone fluids and ion fluxes between interstitial fluid compartments and bone fluids for mineral homeostasis [8]. BLCs show intercellular adhesion molecule 1 while it do not express osteocalcin. These are two important phenotypic differences between BLC and osteoblasts.

1.4 Osteocytes

Osteocytes form more than 90–95% of all the bony cells, whereas osteoblasts and osteoclasts comprise about 4–6% and 1–2% of bone cells, respectively, in an adult skeleton. These are sporadically distributed along the whole mineralized matrix. Their cell body is encapsulated in a structure called lacuna and is connected with each other via dendritic process which traverses bone in a microscopic canal-like structure called canaliculi having dimensions of 250–300 nm [9].

Osteocytes display a distinct morphology both in vivo and in culture that is determined via the expression of E11/PDPN/GP38, PLS3, or CD44. These genes are also expressed in neurons. Osteocytes are now considered as the mechanosensory cells. They have a long lifespan and are found throughout the volume of the bone. Osteocytes give rise to proteins like sclerostin and RANKL, and OPG may influence on other bony cells via autocrine or paracrine pathways. All these happen because of hormonal and mechanical signaling [10].

1.5 Osteocyte formation

Osteocytes arise through the differentiation of osteoblast from the lineage of mesenchymal cells. Four different phases of this process involving (a) osteoid-osteocyte, (b) pre-osteocyte, (c) young osteocyte, and (d) mature osteocyte have been proposed. When the cycle of bone synthesis ends, some osteoblasts' group may be converted into osteocyte embodied in the matrix of bone.

During this process, some notable configurational changes also occur, and this may include reduction in protein production or synthesis and also decrease in round osteoblast shape, which may be correlated with decrease in some organelle count [6].

Furthermore, these cells create a network among them by connecting with nearby osteocytes through many different kinds of lengthy procedures. The network called the lacunar-canalicular network promotes the exchange of nutrients and waste products between osteocytes and acts as a gap junction for communication. Their cell body is deeply present in lacuna, and with the help of canaliculi, their processes arrives to the surrounding osteocytes, and its supply is maintained by Haversian canals through which small vessels move (**Figure 3**) [7].

These cells serve as mechanosensors by means of this system as their connected network can detect mechanical loads applied on bone. This enables the bone to withstand stresses of daily life. Osteocytes also regulate remodeling by controlling the functions of osteoblasts and osteoclasts. Furthermore, it has been established that osteocyte death acts as a stimulus of bone resorption via osteoclasts [6].

Osteocytes detect microfractures in the mineralized bone that result from the mechanical force placed on the bone during movement. In response to this, the cells activate the remodeling process that fix the damaged bone. Osteocytes also detect metabolic signals in addition to the mechanical ones. Aging and estrogen withdrawal, which are linked with increase in bone remodeling and decreased bone mass, increase the risk of their death. Osteocytes in two ways affect osteoblasts: first, they upregulate osteoblasts by producing messengers such as prostaglandin E2 and nitric oxide, and second, they downregulate osteoblasts by releasing sclerostin [11].

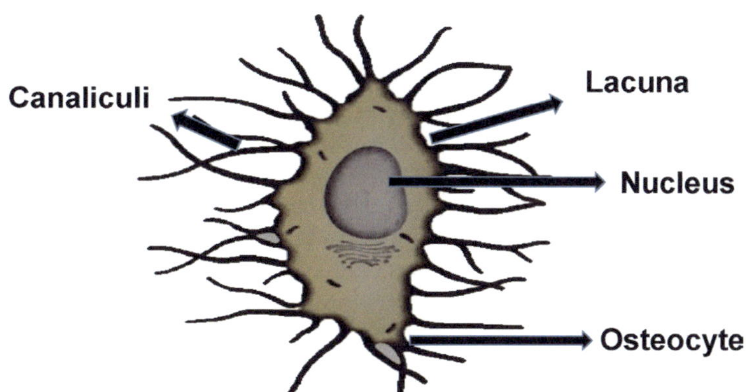

Figure 3.
Osteocyte with its lacuna, a structure containing osteocyte and canaliculi which connect one cell with another through various channels and allow them to exchange their nutrients and transmission of signals necessary for remodeling and repair of bone.

1.6 Osteoclasts

The main cells which are involved in the breakdown of bones are osteoclasts. This role is essential for the maintenance, remodeling, and repair of the vertebral skeleton bones. Human osteoclast gigantic multinucleated entity is 150–200 μm in diameter and typically comprises four nuclei. The transformation of macrophages to osteoclasts by osteoclast-inducing cytokines leads to very massive cells, up to 100 μm in diameter. They may contain dozens of nuclei and express typically major osteoclast proteins, but because of the non-natural substrate, they differ greatly from the other cells that live in bone. The multinucleated constructed osteoclast's size allows it to focus many macrophages' vesicular, protein secretory, and ion transport capacities on a specific region of the bone. The bone multicellular units (BMU) that reshape the bone involves combined activities of osteoblasts, that build bone, and osteoclasts, that break down bone [12]. When osteoclast activity is dysregulated, bony mass rises. Osteoclast precursors stick on osteons' surface and continue to divide, differentiate, and fuse to mature polynucleated entities to initiate bone remodeling. In order that the osteoclast adheres to the bony surface, it disintegrates the matrix loaded with minerals and runs across bony surface and causes certain active domain development. Each osteoclast undergoes programmed cell death (apoptosis) at the completion of bone resorption.

Unlike the cells that we have seen so far, osteoclasts come from HSCs instead of MSCs [7]. Various factors are important in differentiation and survival of osteoclast precursor including RANKL and CSF-1.

Osteoprotegerins inhibit their actions on RANK receptor. The degree of osteoclast development and function is determined by the RANKL/OPG expression ratio. Osteoclast development depends on signaling through mononuclear precursor cell colony stimulating factor receptor. This signaling then upregulates the secretion of RANK and regulates the key osteoclast gene. These genes are required for both the smooth functioning of mature multinucleated osteoclasts and the maturation of osteoclast precursors. In inflammatory diseases like rheumatoid arthritis (RA), pro-inflammatory cytokines and RANKL work in conjunction to stimulate osteoclast formation that is further enhanced by the conversion of dendritic cells into osteoclasts.

Osteoclasts which are mature and non-polarized become activated and are attached to the matrix of bone to cause the resorption. Osteoclasts become polarized when they bind to bone. After adhering to the bone matrix, different kinds of podosomes and domains are formed by the polarized osteoclast.

Podosomes have an actin base encircled by a ring complex consisting of some integrins and cytoskeletal proteins while domains contain SZ, RF, and active secretory domains. After the formation of a ruffle border, some vesicles are shifted toward the membrane via tiny tubules. These vesicles contain cathepsin K and metalloproteinases. At the ruffled border, various enzymes, including cathepsin K, are exocytosed. When the osteoclast's fibrillar actin cytoskeleton come in contact with the bone matrix, an actin ring develops. This creates SZ that separates the surrounding bone surface from the acidified resorption compartment. Bone resorption becomes impeded if either the RB or the SZ is disrupted.

Osteocytes endocytose the fragments of degraded collagen which release the Ca^{2+} and P which are then released at FSD prior to entering the blood stream. Proteolytic enzymes like cathepsin K additionally break down the collagen fragments during this transcytosis process. Small GTPases regulate every stage in the resorption of bone (**Figure 4**) [11].

Microscopic analysis of osteoclasts show that a small, specialized surface of the osteoclast is responsible for resorption. The entire arrangement provides a sealed area where

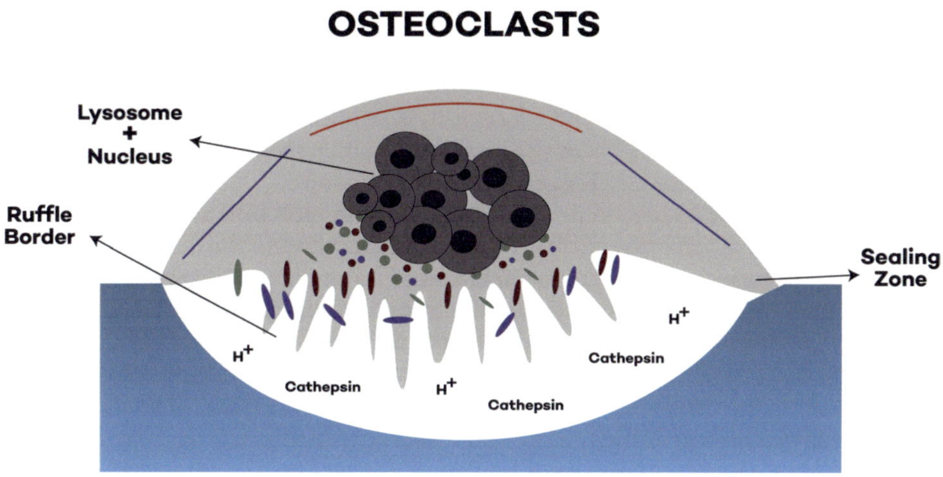

Figure 4.
Osteoclast with their ruffled border and sealing zone and the vesicles that contain H+ and cathepsin moving toward the membrane. This entire arrangement is a sealed area where resorption occurs.

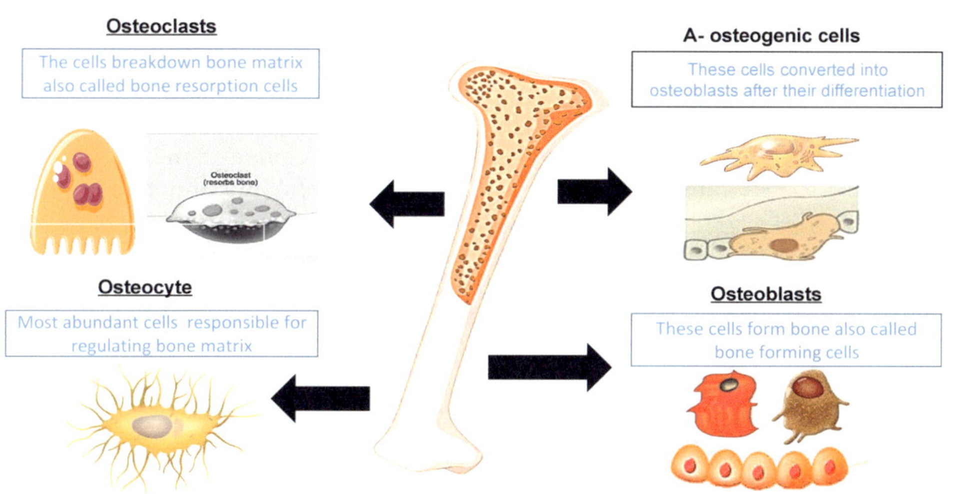

Figure 5.
A visual overview of bone cells that are responsible for the formation of bone and its metabolism, remodeling, and repair, including osteoblasts, osteoclasts, osteocytes, and osteogenic cells with their significant features.

resorption occurs. This enclosed region holds lysosomal contents. The pH is around 4, which is acidic and optimum for lysosomal enzyme to break the bone matrix [5].

Several hormones, that is, calcitonin and PTH, and growth factors such as IL-6 regulate osteoclasts. One contributing element to the condition of 'osteoporosis' is the last hormone, IL-6. Two molecules that are generated by osteoblasts, osteoprotegerin and RANK ligand, interact to influence osteoclast activity as well. These chemicals additionally regulate osteoclast differentiation (**Figure 5**) [12].

There are four different kinds of cells in bone tissue. Osteoblasts are formed by undifferentiated osteogenic cells. Osteoblasts deposit in the bone matrix. When osteoblasts get stuck in the calcified matrix, osteocytes form. Osteoclasts are the particular kind of cell lineage that performs the job of bone resorption (**Table A1**).

1.7 Bone matrix

Bone matrix comprises two components: organic and inorganic. Around 20% of bone mass is made up of organic matrix, mainly composed of collagen. Among them collagen type 1 accounts for 90% of the total bone matrix having less quantity of collagen type III, V, X, and XII (**Figure A1**).

Collagen is a highly branched protein made up of about 1,000 amino acids, organized into a rope-like structure. Collagen provides pliability to the bone; meanwhile, rigidity of the bone is provided by the inclusion of minerals to collagen. If collagen does not contain additional minerals tissues of bone, it will become extremely pliable and possess qualities comparable to a rubber band.

In addition to collagen, proteoglycans and non-collagenous proteins constitute a minor portion (approximately 10%) of the organic matrix's bulk. These include mainly BSP and osteopontin [13].

The main inorganic components of bone include calcium and phosphate ions. Bone matrix has complex and well-organized framework that perform a crucial role in maintaining bone's homeostasis by providing mechanical support. The release of different molecules from the bone matrix may cause the disruption of function of bony cells that leads to bone remodeling [6].

2. The bone remodelling process

Bone undergoes remodeling continuously during the course of an individual's life. In order to maintain structural integrity and metabolic function, bone remodeling is crucial. The remodeling cycle comprises five coordinated steps that takes place within the basic multicellular unit and occurs at different places across the skeleton, simultaneously yet asynchronously. This process involves both local and systemic regulation through various kinds of hormones and growth factors along with some pathways such as canonical Wnt signaling and RANKL/OPG. In vertebrates, the bone performs a variety of functions, such as providing structural support for muscles, storing and releasing growth hormones stored in the matrix, and protecting vital organs and hematopoietic marrow activity [14]. The bone uses its cellular machinery to modify its structural design and material composition to respond various loads [15]. Processes of "construction" and "reconstruction" that occur in bones throughout the life are "bone modeling" and "bone remodeling." In modeling, major changes in the bone structure is brought about through a separate process in which bone resorption and formation occur at different sites on a skeleton. However, in remodeling resorption and formation are closely correlated to one another both spatially and temporally, maintaining the same volume and structure of the bone [16].

- A structure called BMU where both bone cells, that is, OB and OC work together during this process; however, its organization differ in different bones. This implies that cortical bone undergoes approximately 2–5% of remodeling per year.

- This structure creates a canal which is cylindrical in shape, 1000 μm in length and 150–200 μm in width in the cortical bone. A circular tunnel is formed by 10 osteoclasts in the dominant loading direction during a cycle, and multiple osteoblasts fill this. This implies that about 2–5% undergoes remodeling every year.

DOI: http://dx.doi.org/10.5772/intechopen.1005118

- The remodeling is more active in trabecular bone than cortical bone as it has a significantly greater surface to volume ratio. Osteoclasts dig a trench approximately 40–60 m deep by travelling at a speed of around 25 m/day across the trabecular surface [17].

- Bone modeling and remodeling maximize bone strength while reducing mass to satisfy loading and mobility requirements. Where bone is needed, it is deposited by bone formation; where it is not, it is eliminated by bone resorption. Bone modeling mostly takes place during growth.

- It depends on surface of bone, mostly affecting the three inner surface components of the bone, and it is quite less common on the outer bone surface [15].

- Activation, resorption, reversal, formation, and termination are the five stages of bone remodeling cycle. This cycle takes place over several weeks. Bone-lining cells encircle each BMU, providing a unique setting for coupled resorption-formation. The overall size and volume of the bone remains constant during physiological bone remodeling [11].

2.1 Bone modeling

Modeling initiates in early skeletal development in which bone formation and resorption are non-parallel causing changes in the configuration of bone [16]. This process is in contrast with the remodeling process in which bone cell activity is synchronized and happens on particular bony surfaces, while in modeling activity it is unsynchronized or uncoupled and occurs on different sites [18]. This process is done by various drifts that change bones' shape by adding or removing bone tissue from an existing surface to withstand mechanical loads [13]. To achieve this, both OB and OC work separately from each other in space. There are two types of modeling: formation and resorption modeling. Both are done by OB and OC, respectively, having a principal objective of changing the shapes of bones and increasing their mass [18].

When these mechanisms are disrupted, as in the case of *infantile osteogenesis imperfecta* treated with antiresorptive drugs (bisphosphonates), inhibition of this process at metaphysis may occur and exaggerated at diaphysis. In this case, the overall diameter increases with age. Although most bone modeling is finished by when the skeleton reaches adulthood, modeling may still happen in some situations, like during exercise and stress or renal bone disease (**Figure 6**) [16].

2.1.1 Events that signal modeling

Local tissue strain initiates bone modeling. Bone is formed when these stresses are above normal, and formation modeling may occur. Bone is removed, and resorptive modeling begins if stresses are minimal.

The bone cells that detect and respond to mechanical stress are called osteocytes. By the canaliculli, fluid ebbs and flows through compressive forces. Osteocytes sense fluid movement through a structure that protrudes from their cell membrane and is known as the *primary cilium*. The cilium's movement incites signaling pathways in the osteocyte, which raise cytosolic calcium levels and alter gene expression.

Osteoclasts and osteoblasts can be stimulated by the products of these genes to start the process of bone molding. A rise in cytosolic calcium in a single osteocyte may

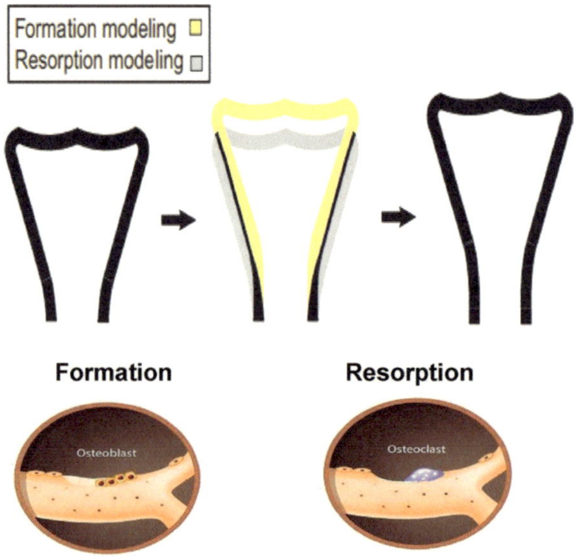

Figure 6.
Bone modelling with the help of osteoblasts and osteoclasts that gives the bone strength to withstand stresses. Yellow color indicates bone formation modeling because of the activity of osteoblast, and grey color represents resorption modeling by the activity of osteoclasts.

spread to other osteocytes because osteocytes are linked by gap junctions. There are two stages of the modeling process: activation and either formation or resorption.

In addition, the stimulation of bone lining cells to differentiate into mature, functional osteoblasts begin forming a matrix. When an adequate quantity of bone mass is added to bear the stress, this process terminates [18].

2.1.2 Bone remodeling

The remodeling process involves bony reconstruction by eliminating discrete, measurable "packets" of bone and replacing them with fresh bone. This happens continuously throughout life, resulting in the growing, adult, and senescent skeletons' ongoing the remodeling of bone [13].

For sufficient physiological bone remodeling to be achieved, proper coupling of formation and resorption is necessary. This is done via direct communication of various bone cells and occurs in a structure called BMU. This structure plays an important role in facilitating this cycle [19].

The BMU is different in its composition and arrangement among different bones and is surrounded by different cells that resemble a canopy to form an area where OB and OC are anatomically coupled to cause remodeling which is called BRC [16].

The cycle of bone remodeling occurs over several weeks and comprises five steps: first activation then resorption after that reversal, then creation, and finally termination [11].

2.1.3 Activation

This represents the very first stage in bone remodeling. The bone is in a quiet or quiescent condition before this. The bone receives and detects the initiating remodeling signal. This signal may be mechanical or hormonal.

It is of two types: targeted and non-targeted. Remodeling that happens because of mechanical forces and micro-damage is termed as targeted. On the other hand, non-targeted remodeling, which is not site-specific, happens because of systemic alterations in various hormones. Osteocytes are also capable of recognizing the biological signals resulting from physical forces. When the signal is detected or recognized, the BLCs begin to retract, collagenase disintegrates the inner membrane of bone, and precursors of osteoclasts are drawn from the bloodstream and are activated.

After their activation, these began to differentiate and start secreting H^+ and several enzymes that initiate the resorption of the bony matrix. When serum calcium levels drop, the parathyroid gland secretes PTH to keep normal homeostasis. It affects the kidneys and bones directly and also the intestines indirectly. This hormone promotes RANKL or MSCF expression to promote osteoclast activation and differentiation by attaching at their receptor site on OB and bone's stromal cells. Additionally, estrogen inhibits the synthesis of RANKL by osteoblasts and osteocytes while concurrently producing OPG from these cells, which decreases the formation of osteoclasts. Thus, as estrogen levels drop among women after menopause, osteoclast survival and production rises, leading to an increase in bone resorption [20–23].

2.1.4 Resorption

During each remodeling cycle, osteoclast-mediated bone resorption lasts approximately about two to four weeks. The cytoskeleton of osteoclasts is reorganized, leading to adhesion to the surface of the bone. Bone OC cells pump proton H^+ in the compartment which is formed by the creation of SZ and RF to increase the area where this secretory activity takes place. This results in the destruction of bone minerals.

Various other enzymes are also released to cleave minerals of bone, and this includes metalloprotease or cat K etc. This leads to the formation of cavities on the surface of trabecular bone that are referred to as Howship's lacunae. The resorption phase is then terminated by the multinucleated osteoclasts undergoing apoptosis [11, 13, 16, 24].

2.1.5 Reversal

We still are not entirely familiar with the reversal phase, which is when bone resorption transforms into formation and lasts approximately four to five weeks. Two major events are believed to be taking place, though. First, the new bone matrix is deposited onto the freshly resorbed bone surface, and further signaling takes place to couple resorption to the formation and prevent net bone loss.

Several coupling signals have been postulated, including the substances generated from the bone matrix, that is, TGF-β whose quantity is equated with markers of turnover in the matrix of bone-like type 1 collagen pro-peptide as well as serum OC. TGF-β reduces osteoclastic resorption by inhibiting osteoblasts from producing RANKL.

Theories suggest that, with their surface regulating receptor and cytokines, osteoclast is the primary source of the factors that are responsible for coupling. Some other factors also included in this are IGF BMP-2 and TGF-b [11, 13, 16, 24].

2.1.6 Formation

The process of bone formation might take four to six months. Osteoblasts form the new, proteinaceous matrix to fill up the cavities that osteoclasts left behind [11].

Several potential coupling mechanisms have been suggested, such as the cell-anchored EphB4ephrin-B2 bidirectional signaling complex and the soluble chemical sphingosine 1-phosphate. Lyso-sphingolipids (S1P) are released by OC which prompts OB precursors' enlistment and increases their survival. Osteoblasts demonstrate EphB4 receptors, while osteoclasts express the ligand Ephrin-B2 that increases osteogenic differentiation by forward signaling.

Both processes of stimulating creation and inhibiting the resorption of bone are achieved by this signaling (eph/ephrin). As a result, coupling may need to occur through a variety of different processes, including soluble signals and direct contact. When osteocytes are at rest, they inhibit bone growth by terminating the Wnt signaling via sclerostin, but when stress is applied, they activate PTH signaling which then promotes bone growth by inhibiting their sclerostin action and maintaining BMD of bone but is still unclear how PTH signaling and mechanical strain interact to enhance remodeling.

MSCs may undergo differentiation to form new bone when MSCs along with OB progenitor cells move toward resorption lacunae. Type 1 collagen is the primary organic substance which makes up bone along with other organic substances and protein as discussed earlier; however, this freshly deposited osteoid is amalgamated by hydroxylapatite [25]

The complex procedure of bone mineralization, that includes the deposition of hydroxyapatite crystals among collagen fibrils, is poorly understood. The ratio of PPi to P is the major regulator in bone mineralization which is affected by a number of factors. Here, PPi is called inorganic pyro-phosphate, and P represents phosphate. Between 50% and 70% of osteoblasts undergo apoptosis after the completion of bone formation, and the remaining osteoblasts convert into osteocytes, or bone-lining cells [11, 13, 16, 20].

2.1.7 Termination

The final stage, which initiates after one month of formation of osteoids, is known as mineralization or calcification and ends after 3 months in trabecular and 120–130 days in cortical bone after the formation of this osteoid. The remodeling cycle is complete when a comparable volume of bone is regained that is being resorbed (**Figure** 7) [11, 16, 25].

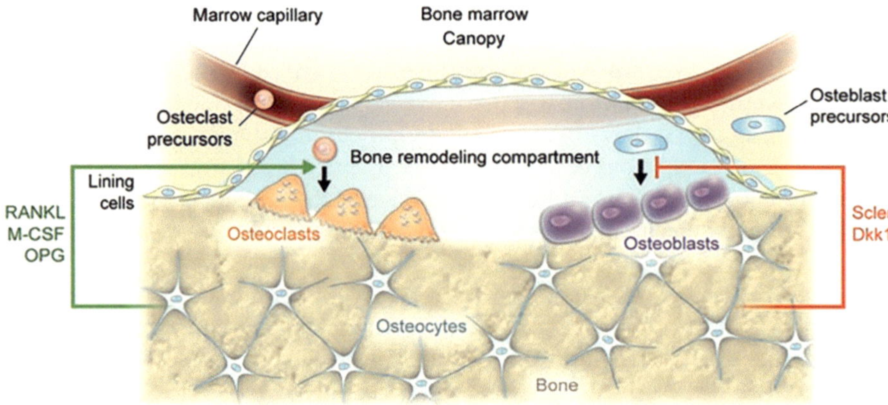

Figure 7.
Bone remodeling compartment: the adjacent bone lining cells receive signals from osteocytes through the canalicular network when bone remodeling is required. After that, a compartment is created where this process occurs by shrinking of these cells called as BRC [24].

The bone remodeling cycle begins when pre-OC comes in contact with bone marrow capillaries and differentiate into mature osteoclasts under the action of pro-osteoclastogenic cytokines derived from osteocytes, such as M-CSF and RANKL. Pre-osteoclasts are pulled in this compartment BRC in which they are converted into OB that forms bone and load up lacuna. This process is believed to be induced by signals derived from osteocytes.

3. Endocrine regulation of bone remodeling

3.1 Parathyroid hormone (PTH)

Parathyroid glands release a polypeptide hormone from their main cells that serves to raise blood calcium levels. PTH affects the kidney and bone directly, and it also indirectly affects the intestines by the action of vitamin D. Furthermore, PTH regulates bone mass in an endocrine way [17, 19, 26].

Depending upon the length of exposure, PTH might have a directly opposing impact on remodeling. Loss of bone mass in both cortical and trabecular bone is because of continuous PTH, whereas cortical bone loss is more severe. The alterations in the OPG-RANKL-RANK signaling pathway by PTH are responsible for these catabolic consequences. Osteocytes and osteoblasts are the source of continuous PTH, which stimulates osteoclastogenesis by inhibiting OPG and increasing RANKL [26].

Lower plasma calcium concentrations activate the negative feedback process and cause less binding to the parathyroid gland's calcium-sensing receptors (CaSR). As a result, more PTH will be released, increasing the levels of calcium. This hormone also affects OC indirectly by increasing RANKL activity which controls their action and results in more plasma calcium levels.

On the other hand, binding to the CASR receptor is lessened when the plasma calcium concentration is increased and this will inhibit PTH release. When CaSRs are stimulated, the receptor undergoes a conformational shift that stimulates the phospholipase C pathway. This eventually results in increased intracellular calcium that inhibits PTH from being exocytosed from the parathyroid gland's chief cells.

On the other hand, to treat osteoporosis, PTH is administered intermittently and acts as an anabolic agent. Sclerostin along with dickkopf-1 are expressed less when PTH signaling is intermittent, whereas Wnt ligand Wnt10b is expressed more. Osteoblastogenesis and bone formation increase when canonical Wnt signaling increased [16, 26].

3.2 Estrogen

Estrogen is the primary hormone that regulates bone metabolism in both men and women [27–29].

Estrogens promote the formation of new bone while inhibiting resorption. Men with insufficient levels reconstruct at a faster rate because they produce less estrogen from testosterone by aromatization [16].

In cases of estrogen insufficiency, there is an increase in bone remodeling which causes a reduction in bony mass because resorption is much more than formation [26].

The concept that osteoporosis results from decreased bone formation after menopause was initially proposed by Albright et al. in the 1940s. IL-1 and TNF production suppression is done by estrogen. These are not only well-known inhibitors of formation but also a powerful bone resorption promotor.

They directly affect osteoblast cells, which in turn indirectly activates adult osteoclasts. According to certain studies, TNF and IL-1 stimulate osteoclast precursor activity directly, which increases the production of osteoclast cells. The action of these cytokines is blocked by estrogen. Estrogen indirectly limits IL-6 expression. The actions of TNF and IL-1 that upregulate IL-6 and assist its actions are blocked, and that is why, this happens. IL-6 mainly stimulates the process of osteoclastogenesis by stimulating osteoclast precursors. As estrogen inhibits osteoclastogenesis, it therefore has a bone-protective effect. This hormone activates estrogen osteoprotegerin (OPG) and facilitates mature osteoclast's programmed death directly. This OPG then regulates bony mass [30].

3.3 Calcitonin (CT)

C-cells of the thyroid gland release a hormone called calcitonin in response to elevated calcium levels that inhibit bone resorption by binding to osteoclast's calcitonin receptor, decreasing their number, secretory activity, and formation of ruffled borders [26, 31].

It was also said that the main regulator of bone resorption process is calcitonin. Because of this, calcitonin has been used widely in clinics to treat bone conditions such osteoporosis, hypercalcemia, and Paget's disease [32].

It is also believed that osteoblast-like cells lack calcitonin receptors, but in certain systems, this hormone reacts to OBs and enhances the osteoinduction of rhBMP-2. However, the effects of this hormone are still unclear on osteoblasts [19].

3.4 Thyroid hormone

The relationship between thyroid hormones and bone formation was first understood in the 1890s when von Recklinghausen noted a patient with hyperthyroidism and multiple fractures [33].

Thyroid hormones T_3 and T_4 along with TSH cause expansion of epiphyseal plate of long bones via OB stimulation [26].

Thyroid hormone exerts a significant effect on bone and mineral metabolism and is an important modulator of bone remodeling [34, 35].

About 100 years later, we still know that hyperthyroidism causes a 10% loss of bone by increasing their turnover, slowing or delaying their remodeling process, and uncouples osteoblastic and osteoclastic activity. This might lead to osteoporosis. On the other hand, adolescents with hypothyroidism suffer delayed skeletal development and maturation, epiphyseal dysgenesis, and retarded long bone growth. Adult hypothyroidism has been associated with decreased bone turnover and osteosclerosis; both conditions can be resolved frequently with thyroid hormone therapy [16, 29].

Triiodothyronine (T3), a physiologically active thyroxine derivative, influences both osteoblasts and osteoclasts in vitro. T3 affects osteoblasts in two ways: it has been noticed that it inhibits osteoblast proliferation and promotes osteoblast differentiation in both primary and calvarial osteoblasts and osteoblastic cell lines. In osteoclasts, T3 acts directly or indirectly through cytokines and stimulates osteoclast activity [19].

The thyroid hormone receptors (TR) TRα1 and TRβ1 which are encoded by Thra and Thrb gene, respectively, modulate the actions of TH on bone [35].

3.5 Glucocorticoids

Glucocorticoids have a significant impact on the function, differentiation, and replication of bone cells. They promote bone resorption by increasing the expression of collagenase 3. Glucocorticoids have three main effects on osteoblasts: (a) increase their programmed cell death, (b) decrease their differentiation, and (c) reduce their activity by altering the expression of binding proteins and various growth factors. Glucocorticoids increase the risk of osteoporotic fractures by causing rapid bone loss. In cartilage, these hormones inhibit linear growth by modifying GH and IGF [36].

The bone resorption is largely because of direct actions of glucocorticoids on the skeleton and partially due to an increase in calcium excretion in urine and a decrease in an intestinal absorption of calcium. The mechanism by which glucocorticoids oppose the effects of vitamin D in vivo by inhibiting intestinal calcium transport is still unclear [37].

Secondary hyperparathyroidism has been suggested due to elevated renal calcium losses and decreased absorption of calcium, but in glucocorticoids-induced-osteoporosis, it does not seem to be significant.

It is suspected that increased sensitivity to parathyroid hormone (PTH) contributes to the observed bone resorption. As parathyroid hormone/PTH-related peptide's expression is increased by the glucocorticoids, consistent increase of blood PTH or a pattern of bone loss similar to hyperparathyroidism should be expected if the process results in a hyperparathyroid state that occurs in a glucocorticoid-induced-osteoporosis (GIO). But there is no correlation between the acute or long-term use of glucocorticoids and serum PTH levels in the hyperparathyroidism range. Further evidence from bone densitometry suggests that PTH is not involved in glucocorticoid-induced osteoporosis.

A condition that is recognized by cortical bone loss while cancellous bone is preserved is primary hyperparathyroidism; in contrast, glucocorticoid-induced-osteoporosis (GIO) shows an opposite pattern of preferential bone loss. It is confirmed by histomorphometric investigation of bone biopsies that glucocorticoids-induced-osteoporosis and hyperparathyroidism are two different disorders. Osteoblast number is preserved, but bone turnover is increased in primary hyperparathyroidism.

On the other hand, the turnover of bone along with the loss of OBs occurs in GIO. These explanations suggest that PTH do not prominently cause glucocorticoid-induced osteoporosis. When pre-osteoclasts' RANK receptors are stimulated by the attachment of RANKL, it in association with CSF-1 prompts osteoclastogenesis.

In order to prevent osteoclast receptor from attaching the RANKL, osteoprotegerin binds to RANKL and functions as a decoy receptor. RANKL and CSF1 expressions are upregulated by glucocorticoids, but osteoprotegerin expression is downregulated in the surrounding stromal cells and osteoblasts. Consequently, there is an increase in the production of osteoclasts and bone resorption [26, 36].

When exposed to glucocorticoids, bone resorption is inhibited by bisphosphonate, which also stops and reverses bone loss. But evidence from clinical setting states that people with GIO have bone loss in the starting months when they are exposed to glucocorticoids. Anabolic substances can enhance bone mass in the GIO by promoting bone formation, such as parathyroid hormone [36–38].

3.6 Growth hormone and IGF

Growth hormone is released from anterior pituitary gland under hypothalamic regulation. It plays multiple roles in the human body, including control of several metabolic pathways, regulating the release and the function of other hormones, and interacting with the immune system. But as its name suggests, the most studied task it performs is coordinating longitudinal growth. Through the local and systemic synthesis of IGF-I, GH affects directly as well as indirectly. As the development and metabolism of bone is controlled via both GH and IGF-I, they also influence bone mass. Throughout childhood, bone mass gradually grows, reaching a peak in the middle of 20s. There is a consequent gradual decrease that quickens at later age.

In childhood, both growth and remodeling causes bone mass development. In order to promote bone formation, GH both directly and indirectly increases osteoblast proliferation and activity through IGF-I. It has been found that osteoblastic MC3T3-E1 cells have GH binding sites [39].

In addition to that, it also increases osteoclast activity and differentiation which promotes bone resorption. As a result, there is a net increase in bone accumulation and raise in the overall momentum of the remodeling process. When GH lacks, bone remodeling occurs more slowly and eventually loses bone mineral density. Although GH directly affects chondrocytes, it mostly controls their function by stimulating the formation of matrix and cell proliferation in these cells through IGF-I [26, 40, 41].

A long-term GH therapy may reverse the severe limitation on bone growth and a decrease in bone mineral density caused by GH deficiency [42].

4. Bone growth or ossification

A process that begins at 6–7th week of embryogenesis and goes till the age of 25, in which bone formation occurs, is known as ossification or osteogenesis of bone. This process varies in different individuals and in different bones [43].

There are two types of bone ossification: intramembranous and endochondral ossification. In both cases, pre-existing mesenchymal tissue is converted into bone tissue. Intramembranous ossification refers to the process of directly converting mesenchymal tissue into bone to form flat bones. This procedure primarily occurs in the skull's bones. On the other hand, the mesenchymal cells may develop into cartilage, which is then converted to bone [44].

4.1 Intramembranous ossification

This process does not begin with an existing cartilage model. Intramembranous ossification is the process through which most of the skull's bones and a few other (flat) bones, including the clavicle and scapula, forms embryonically. Intramembranous ossification begins in mesenchyme, which is embryonic connective tissue having mesenchymal cells. This typically is linked to embryonic development, and intramembranous ossification may also occur after birth (during bone repair or healing). During their first stage, a blastema is formed which is made by the combination of the mesenchymal cells. This produces bone matrix after their OB differentiation. To direct their cells toward the osteoblastic lineage, RUNX plays a key role.

The process in which formation of bone takes place within a particular area is known as the primary ossification center, which is established when osteoblasts produces the initial bone matrix. Thus, more and more matrix is produced, and few osteoblasts get encapsulated and transform into osteocytes.

Woven bone is formed by initial OBs. More osteoblasts are drawn to the surface, where they continue to produce this bone and then lamellar bone and continue to form the matrix until the required matrix is formed. Some bones, during development, may form as a result of the union of many tiny bony islands. In some bones, including the jaw, that is formed by the intramembranous ossification, there is the creation of some cavities to allow vessels to invade the ossification core (**Figure 8**) [18, 24].

4.2 Endochondral ossification

A process by which majority of bones, that is, skull base bones (including ethmoid and sphenoid bone), the axial (ribs and vertebrae) and the appendicular bones, long bones, the medial end of the clavicle, as well as short bones are developed is called endochondral ossification [21].

Shrinking of mesenchymal cells, similar to intramembranous ossification, starts this process. These cells differentiate into chondroblasts rather than of osteoblasts. SOX-9 is the transcription factor that drives this process. These cells, called chondroblasts, create a matrix of cartilage that eventually surrounds certain other cells, converting them into chondrocytes. The perichondrium surrounds the hyaline cartilage. Osteoblastic differentiation occurs on this cartilage and initiates building the

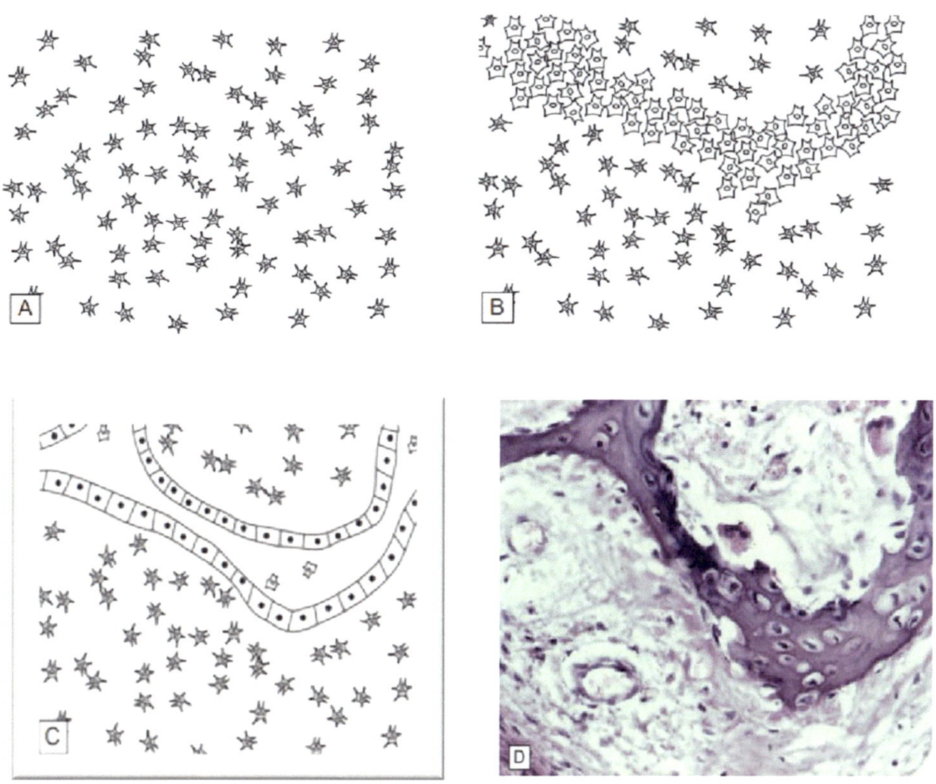

Figure 8.
The intramembranous ossification taking place in the sea of mesenchymal cells. (A) In the beginning, mesenchymal stem cells assemble into blastema and convert into osteoblasts. (B) Production of bone matrix. (C) Bone matrix undergoing remodeling. (D) Photomicrograph showing the jaw's intramembranous ossification-forming island of bone (eosin and hematoxylin stain) [18, 20].

bone. The transcription factor RUNX2 controls this osteoblast differentiation process, much like it does during intramembranous ossification. The long bone's diaphysis, or midshaft, is where bone growth first takes place, giving rise to a structure known as the bone collar.

After the formation of this structure, calcification of matrix occurs because the cartilage cells die. Through the osteoclast assistance, there is the entry of primary blood vessel via this collar, in the area of calcified cartilage. These vessels help in the transportation of osteoclasts which not only provide nutrients for remaining cells but also form the primary ossification center [18]. Primary and secondary sites are two different locations where this process takes place, and among them, the bone initially grows at the primary site. After that, growth at epiphyseal plate occurs which is responsible for longitudinal growth. This process involves five steps [22].

4.2.1 Zones of endochondral ossification

4.2.1.1 Resting zone

The resting zone is the furthest region from cartilage template's margins composed of chondrocytes embedded in the hyaline cartilage matrix. At some places, this zone is named as the reverse zone [23].

The chondroblasts adjacent to the perichondrium continually generate new resting zone matrix that is rich in type II collagen. The chondrocytes however are embedded in the matrix to generate a new matrix. Both morphological and physiological properties of the chondrocytes in the resting zone are similar to those of hyaline cartilage in other body parts.

4.2.1.2 Proliferative zone

As the name suggests, the proliferative zone, which is the second area, is the place of active chondrocyte mitosis as shown in **Figure 9**. The stacked coin appearance of this region is the result of the longitudinal division of cells which makes it readily identifiable histologically. These cells produce significant amounts of type II collagen-rich matrix. Various growth factors, signaling pathways, and proteins regulate the zone of proliferation. Some of these are somatotropin, IHH, IGFs, and BMPs. Among few substances that has been demonstrated to stop chondrocyte proliferation in this region is fibroblast growth factor (FGF).

4.2.1.3 Hypertrophic zone

It is the third zone in which cells are arranged in two portions; among them, lower zone's cells continue to grow and undergo death, while higher zone's cells cause long bone growth. Thyroxine along with Wnt-b-catenin pathways is responsible for increase in cartilage cell's size, while PTHrP and IHH inhibit hypertrophy of cartilage cells. This hypertrophy causes the cell to grow and synthesize matrix that is rich in type 2 collagen. However, this area also exhibits a shift in type II collagen production to type X collagen. Genetic programs lead to a sharp increase in chondrocyte cell size, a shift in production of type 2 toward COL10A1, and the induction of substance like VEGF and ALP that causes the cartilage matrix to calcify and vascularize all components of hypertrophic differentiation [45].

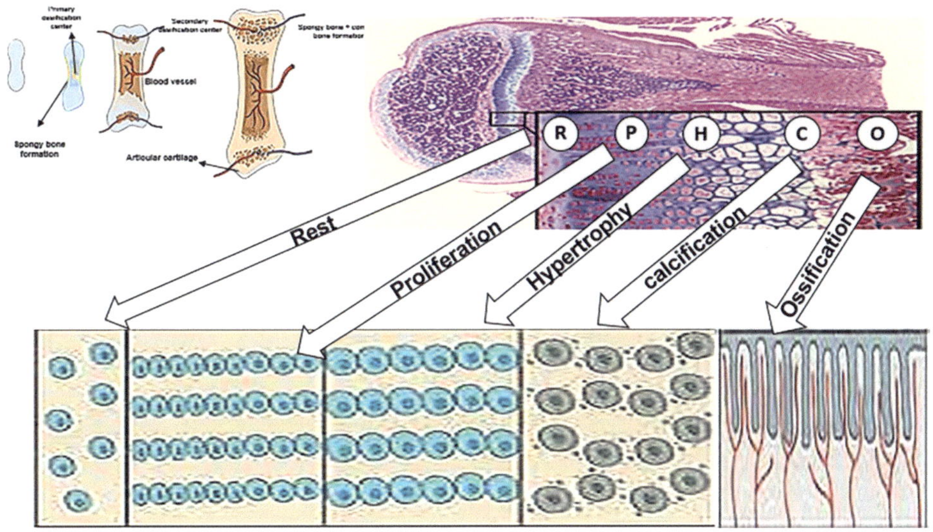

Figure 9.
Endochondral ossification of bones cells passing through different phases of resting zone, proliferative zone, hypertrophy zone, calcification, and ossification zone to convert the cartilage template into bone to facilitate the growth of bone.

4.2.1.4 Zone of calcification

It is the stage where cartilage calcification is observable. Because of inadequate cellular waste removal or nutrient diffusion, the cells of the cartilage may die in this zone.

4.2.1.5 Zone of ossification

The zone of ossification is the last zone, where bone initially forms. Toward this calcified tissue surface, osteoblasts are drawn from the skeletal tissue to build woven bone.

Osteoblasts that are recruited to the surface of calcified tissue (to form new woven bone) form the skeletal tissue. Osteoclasts also exist in the ossification zone and act to remove calcified cartilage as well as newly formed woven bone, which is through remodeling subsequently converted into lamellar bone (**Figure 9**) [18].

Acknowledgements

We would like to express our gratitude to the authors from the Department of Physical Therapy at Islamia University of Bahawalpur, the Department of Medical Laboratory Technology at Islamia University Bahawalpur, and Quaid-e-Azam Medical College, Bahawalpur, for their contributions to the writing, editing, and analysis of this paper.

Conflict of interest

The authors declare no conflict of interest.

Abbreviations

MSCs	mesenchymal stem cells
BMPs	bone morphogenic proteins
BMU	basis multicellular unit
HSCs	hematopoietic stem cells
Sz	sealing zone
Rf	ruffled border
FSD	functional secreting domain
CATK	cathepsin k
BLCs	bone lining cells
BRC	bone remodeling compartment

A. Appendix

Cell type	Function	Location
Osteogenic cells	Develop in osteoblast	Deep layers of periosteum and the marrow
Osteoblast	Bone formation	Growing portion of bone including periosteum and endosteum
Osteocytes	Maintain matrix mineral concentration	Entrapped in matrix
Osteoclasts	Bone resorption	Bone surfaces and at sites of old, injured, or unneeded bone

Table A1.
Bone cells along with their functions and location.

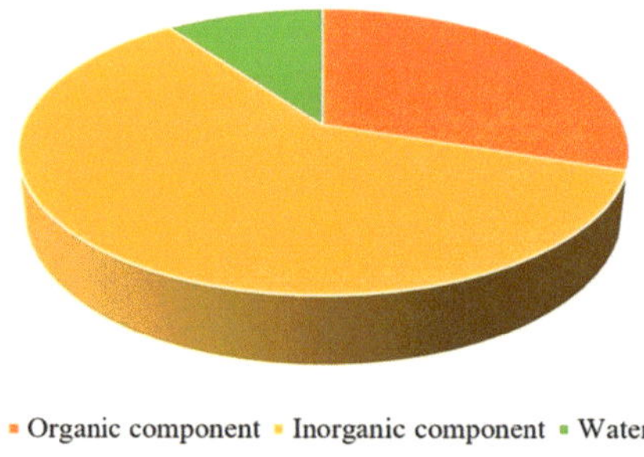

Figure A1.
Components that form bone matrix. Inorganic components consititute the most part [9].

B. Osteoblasts

Some of the osteoblasts possess cytoplasmic projections travel in bone matrix direction and finally reached to osteocyte process. At this stage, this OB has two choices: either they are converted into osteocyte or BLCs or undergo programmed cell death. Surprisingly, in the vacuoles of osteoblasts, there are some ovoid bodies having dense bodies, and some TUNEL-positive structures are found. These finding indicate that they are also able to engulf apoptotic material in an addition to skilled phagocytosis during alveolar development of bone [12, 14].

C. Bone lining cells

Recent studies suggest that bone lining cells anchored the hematopoitic stem cells that gives stimulus to them to remain in their undifferentiated state. These cells play a crucial role in changes that are associated with the bone remodeling promoting HSCs differentiation toward osteoclasts and by using matrix metaloproteinases. These cells prepare bone surface by excluding the unmineralized collagen fibril. During their transformation from osteoblasts to osteocytes, some proteins that form phenotype of osteoblast are no longer produced. These include alkaline phosphatases, collagen type 1 osteocalcin, and bone sialoprotein [15].

D. Osteoclasts

Based on electron micrographs, membrane part that is nearest to the mineralized bone surface is highly convoluted and forms ruffled border. A membrane ring called as the sealing zone, seals the resorption area by tightly connecting to the bone and, is present at the outer edge of the ruffled border. And, it is a site where the osteoclast attaches to the surface of bone and where the actual bone resorption occurs. It is also the site where the osteoclast secretes acid (protons H^+), which acidifies the surrounding environment and other lysosomal enzymes, such as cathepsin K, which breaks down the organic components of the bone matrix.

E. Bone matrix

Collagen is a fibrous highly convoluted protein consisting of thousands of amino acids. These are arranged into a rope-like structure which is 300 nm in length. Its fibrils are made up of one $\alpha 2$ and two $\alpha 1$ polypeptide chains that assemble to form triple helical procollagen molecule inside OBs. These osteoblasts release the pro collagen molecules causing the assembling of each collagen molecule to form collagen fibril which then together forms collagen fiber.

Without collagen, bone becomes brittle just like a chalk. Various processes and abnormalities including aging and genetics can influence its structure, affect structural integrity of bone tissue, and cause weakening of it and become more prone to fracture than normal.

Proteoglycans and non-collagenous proteins form a minor portion of the organic matrix's bulk, but they are essential for osteoblast differentiation, tissue mineralization, cell adhesion, and bone remodeling [25].

A minute concentration of bicarbonate, sodium, potassium, citrate, magnesium, carbonate, fluorite, zinc, barium, and strontium also constitute inorganic component in addition to calcium and phosphate. Hydroxyapatite crystals, that have a chemical formula of $Ca_{10}(PO_4)_6(OH)_2$, are formed when calcium and phosphate ions nucleate [14].

F. Bone modeling and remodeling

F.1 Activation

There is active 1,25 vitamin D3 production from inactive precursor and increases calcium absorption by the kidneys because of PTH (**Figure A2**). This 1,25 VitD3 influences the resorption of bone indirectly and also increases RANKL and MCSF expression by this. Finally, estrogen's function in the process of bone remodeling is a bone sparing hormone. Both osteoblasts and osteoclasts express estrogen receptors. By causing pre-osteoclast and osteoclast apoptosis, while inhibiting osteoblast and osteocyte apoptosis, and limiting excessive bone resorption, estrogen plays a critical role in controlling the longevity of bone cells [25, 28, 32].

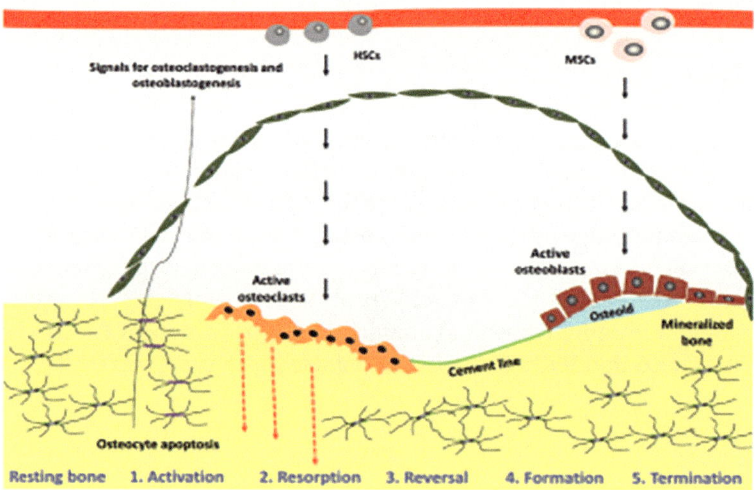

Figure A2.
An Illustration of the various stage of bone remodeling; activation, resorption, reversal, creation and termination in the bone remodeling cycle.

F.2 Ossification

The zone of reserve in which hyaline cartilage acts as a storehouse for chondrocytes may aid in the process of growth. This photomicrograph's zone of proliferation, in which chondrocytes proliferate quickly, is located at the top divide and become stacked in a longitudinal orientation. The zone of hypertrophy in which chondrocytes enlarge and undergo terminal differentiation, and they subsequently compress the matrix into aligned spicules and secrete type X collagen to stiffen it. The zone of calcified cartilage is where chondrocytes release osteocalcin and matrix vesicles that cause the matrix to start to calcify by crystallizing hydroxyapatite. The zone of ossification is where bone tissue initially appears. Here, osteoblasts form a layer over the calcified cartilage matrix's spicules and release osteoid (**Figure A3**), which then develops into woven bone (that further modified into lamellar bone) (**Figure A4**) [46].

DOI: http://dx.doi.org/10.5772/intechopen.1005118

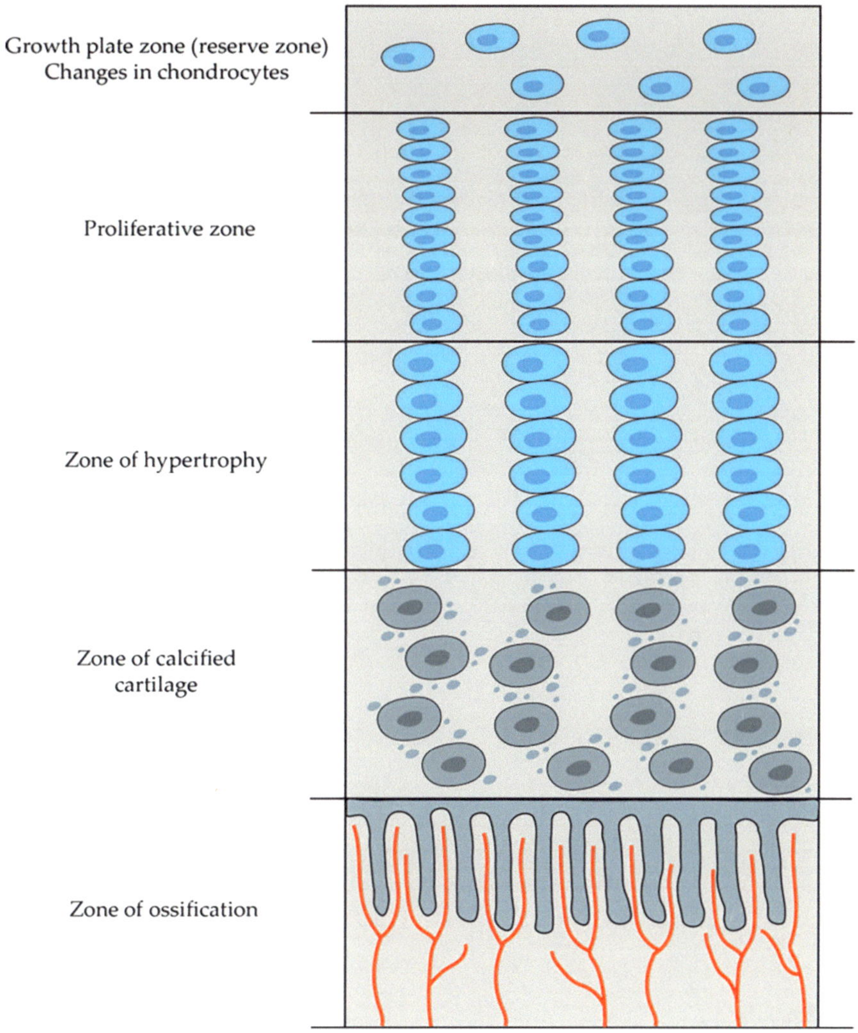

Figures A3.
Various of the endochondral ossification and involved mechanism.

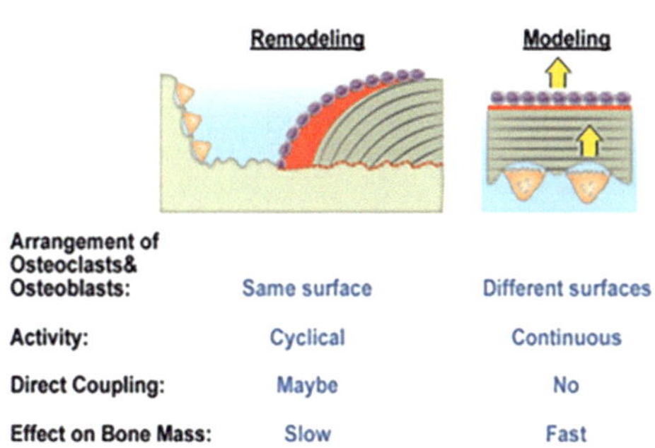

Figures A4.
Remodeling versus modeling: In bone remodeling, the formation of bones and resorption are simultaneously mediated by osteoclasts at the same site. Its main goal are to regenerate the skeleton and recover micor-damage. The periosteal, endocortical, intracortical, and trabecular envelopes all undergoes remodeling. Bone modeling mostlt take placed during skeletal growth.

Author details

Ayesha Bashir[1]*, Qurrat ul Ain[2], Naveeda Bashir[3] and Wajahat Sohail[1]

1 Department of Physical Therapy, Islamia University of Bahawalpur, Pakistan

2 Department of Medical Laboratory Technology, Islamia University of Bahawalpur, Pakistan

3 Quaid e Azam Medical College, Bahawalpur, Pakistan

*Address all correspondence to: ayesha.bashir@iub.edu.pk

References

[1] Setiawati R, Rahardjo P. Bone development and growth. In: Osteogenesis and Bone Regeneration. 2019. pp. 1-10. DOI: 10.5772/intechopen.82452

[2] Su N, Yang J, Xie Y, Du X, Chen H, Zhou H, et al. Bone function, dysfunction and its role in diseases including critical illness. International Journal of Biological Sciences. 2019;**15**(4):776. DOI: 10.7150%2Fijbs.27063

[3] Boskey AL, Robey PG. The composition of bone. In: Primer on the Metabolic Bone Diseases and Disorders of Mineral Metabolism. 8th ed. 2013. pp. 49-58. DOI: 10.1002/9781118453926.ch6

[4] Alghazali KM, Nima ZA, Hamzah RN, Dhar MS, Anderson DE, Biris AS. Bone-tissue engineering: complex tunable structural and biological responses to injury, drug delivery, and cell-based therapies. Drug Metabolism Reviews. 2015;**47**(4):431-454. DOI: 10.3109/03602532.2015.1115871

[5] Rodan GA. Introduction to bone biology. Bone. 1992;**13**:S3-S6. DOI: 10.1016/S8756-3282(09)80003-3

[6] Florencio-Silva R, Sasso GR, Sasso-Cerri E, Simões MJ, Cerri PS. Biology of bone tissue: Structure, function, and factors that influence bone cells. BioMed Research International. 2015;**2015**:1-17. DOI: 10.1155/2015/421746

[7] Brown JL, Laurencin CT. Bone tissue engineering. In: Biomaterials Science. San Diego, United States: Academic Press, Elsevier Inc; 2020. pp. 1373-1388. DOI: 10.1016/B978-0-12-816137-1.00085-4

[8] Miller SC, de Saint-Georges L, Bowman BM, Jee WS. Bone lining cells: structure and function. Scanning Microscopy. 1989;**3**(3):27 Available from: https://pubmed.ncbi.nlm.nih.gov/2694361/

[9] Bonewald LF. Osteocytes. In: Marcus and Feldman's Osteoporosis. Cambridge, Massachusetts, USA: Academic Press, Elsevier; 2021. pp. 135-163. DOI: 10.1016/B978-0-12-813073-5.00007-1

[10] Bellido T, Plotkin LI, Bruzzaniti A. Bone cells. In: Basic and Applied Bone Biology. New York: Academic Press, Elsevier; 2019. pp. 37-55. DOI: 10.1016/B978-0-12-813259-3.00003-8

[11] Katsimbri P. The biology of normal bone remodelling. European Journal of Cancer Care. 2017;**26**(6):e12740. DOI: 10.1111/ecc.12740

[12] Wikipedia Contributors. Osteoclast. In *Wikipedia. The Free Encyclopedia*. 2024. Available from: https://en.wikipedia.org/w/index.php?title=Osteoclast&oldid=1193964632

[13] Fuchs RK, Thompson WR, Warden SJ. Bone biology. In: Bone Repair Biomaterials. United Kingdom: Woodhead Publishing, Elsevier; 2019. pp. 15-52. DOI: 10.1016/B978-0-08-102451-5.00002-0

[14] Boyce BF, Xing L. Functions of RANKL/RANK/OPG in bone modeling and remodeling. Archives of Biochemistry and Biophysics. 2008;**473**(2):139-146. DOI: 10.1016/j.abb.2008.03.018

[15] Seeman E. Bone modeling and remodeling. Critical Reviews™ in Eukaryotic Gene Expression. 2009;**19**(3):219-233. Available from: https://pubmed.ncbi.nlm.nih.gov/19883366/

[16] Kenkre JS, Bassett JH. The bone remodelling cycle. Annals of Clinical Biochemistry. 2018;**55**(3):308-327. DOI: 10.1177/0004563218759371

[17] Hadjidakis DJ, Androulakis II. Bone remodeling. Annals of the New York Academy of Sciences. 2006;**1092**(1):385-396. DOI: 10.1196/annals.1365.035

[18] Allen MR, Burr DB. Bone modeling and remodeling. In: Basic and Applied Bone Biology. London, United Kingdom: Academic Press, Elsevier; 2014. pp. 75-90. DOI: 10.1016/B978-0-12-416015-6.00004-6

[19] Siddiqui JA, Partridge NC. Physiological bone remodeling: Systemic regulation and growth factor involvement. Physiology. 2016;**31**(3):233-245. DOI: 10.1152/physiol.00061.2014

[20] Runyan CM, Gabrick KS. Biology of bone formation, fracture healing, and distraction osteogenesis. The Journal of Craniofacial Surgery. 2017;**28**(5):1380-1389. DOI: 10.1097/SCS.0000000000003625

[21] Wikipedia Contributors. Endochondral ossification. In *Wikipedia, The Free Encyclopedia*. 2024. Available from: https://en.wikipedia.org/w/index.php?title=Endochondral_ossification&oldid=1203087703 [Accessed: 16 July 2024]

[22] Ortega N, Behonick DJ, Werb Z. Matrix remodeling during endochondral ossification. Trends in Cell Biology. 2004;**14**(2):86-93. DOI: 10.1016/j.tcb.2003.12.003

[23] Douglas J. Chapter 54 – Pathogenesis of osteochondrosis. In: Diagnosis and Management of Lameness in the Horse. Vol. 2. USA: Elsevier; 2011. pp. 617-625. DOI: 10.1016/B978-1-4160-6069-7.00054-7

[24] Gasser JA, Kneissel M. Bone physiology and biology. Bone Toxicology. 2017;**1**:27-94. DOI: 10.1007/978-3-319-56192-9_2

[25] Raggatt LJ, Partridge NC. Cellular and molecular mechanisms of bone remodeling. The Journal of Biological Chemistry. 2010;**285**(33):25103-25108. DOI: 10.1074/jbc.R109.041087

[26] Rowe P, Koller A, Sharma S. Physiology, bone remodeling. In: StatPearls. Treasure Island (FL): StatPearls Publishing; 2023. Available from: https://europepmc.org/article/NBK/nbk499863. PMID: 29763038

[27] Cauley JA. Estrogen and bone health in men and women. Steroids. 2015;**99**:11-15. DOI: 10.1016/j.steroids.2014.12.010

[28] Khosla S, Oursler MJ, Monroe DG. Estrogen and the skeleton. Trends in Endocrinology and Metabolism. 2012;**23**(11):576-581. DOI: 10.1016/j.tem.2012.03.008

[29] Noirrit-Esclassan E, Valera MC, Tremollieres F, Arnal JF, Lenfant F, Fontaine C, et al. Critical role of estrogens on bone homeostasis in both male and female: From physiology to medical implications. International Journal of Molecular Sciences. 2021;**22**(4):1568. DOI: 10.3390/ijms22041568

[30] Aayushi B, Kekatpure AL. Postmenopausal osteoporosis: A literature review. Cureus. 2022;**14**(9):1-15. DOI: 10.7759%2Fcureus.29367

[31] Hsiao CY, Chen TH, Chu TH, Ting YN, Tsai PJ, Shyu JF. Calcitonin induces bone formation by increasing expression of Wnt10b in osteoclasts in ovariectomy-induced osteoporotic rats. Frontiers in Endocrinology. 2020;**11**:613. DOI: 10.3389/fendo.2020.00613

[32] Xie J, Guo J, Kanwal Z, Wu M, Lv X, Ibrahim NA, et al. Calcitonin and bone physiology: In vitro, in vivo, and clinical investigations. International Journal of Endocrinology. 2020;**2020**:1-20. DOI: 10.1155/2020/3236828

[33] Altabas V, Berkovic M, Becejac B, Solter M. Bone remodeling and thyroid function. Acta Clinica Croatica. 2007;**46**(1):41 Available from: https://www.researchgate.net/publication/229023185_Bone_remodeling_and_thyroid_function

[34] Mosekilde L, Eriksen EF, Charles P. Effects of thyroid hormones on bone and mineral metabolism. Endocrinology and Metabolism Clinics of North America. 1990;**19**(1):35-63. DOI: 10.1016/S0889-8529(18)30338-4

[35] Lademann F, Tsourdi E, Hofbauer LC, Rauner M. Thyroid hormone receptor Thra and Thrb knockout differentially affects osteoblast biology and thyroid hormone responsiveness in vitro. Journal of Cellular Biochemistry. 2023;**124**(12):1948-1960. DOI: 10.1002/jcb.30500

[36] Canalis E. Mechanisms of glucocorticoid action in bone. Current Osteoporosis Reports. 2005;**3**(3):98-102. DOI: 10.1007/s11914-005-0017-7

[37] Canalis ER. Clinical review 83: Mechanisms of glucocorticoid action in bone: implications to glucocorticoid-induced osteoporosis. The Journal of clinical endocrinology & metabolism. 1996;**81**(10):3441-3447. DOI: 10.1111/j.1749-6632.2002.tb04204.x

[38] Kim HJ, Zhao H, Kitaura H, Bhattacharyya S, Brewer JA, Muglia LJ, et al. Glucocorticoids and the osteoclast. Annals of the New York Academy of Sciences. 2007;**1116**(1):335-339. DOI: 10.1196/annals.1402.057

[39] Chihara K, Sugimoto T. The action of GH/IGF-I/IGFBP in osteoblasts and osteoclasts. Hormone Research. 1997;**48**:45-49. DOI: 10.1159/000191328

[40] Olney RC. Regulation of bone mass by growth hormone. Medical and Pediatric Oncology. 2003;**41**(3):228-234. DOI: 10.1002/mpo.10342

[41] Inzucchi SE, Robbins RJ. Growth hormone and the maintenance of adult bone mineral density. Clinical Endocrinology. 1996;**45**(6):665-673. DOI: 10.1046/j.1365-2265.1996.8750885.x

[42] Ohlsson V. Effects of growth hormone and insulin-like growth factors on human osteoblasts. European Journal of Clinical Investigation. 1998;**28**(3):184-186. DOI: 10.1046/j.1365-2362.1998.00266.x

[43] Breeland G, Sinkler MA, Menezes RG. Embryology, Bone Ossification. Treasure Island, Florida, USA: StatPearls Publishing. Available from: https://www.ncbi.nlm.nih.gov/books/NBK539718/

[44] Gilbert SF. Osteogeesis: The Development of Bones: Developmental Biology. 6th ed. Sunderland, Massachusetts, USA: Sinauer Associates; 2000. Available from: https://www.ncbi.nlm.nih.gov/books/NBK10056/

[45] Karner CM, Hilton MJ. Endochondral ossification. In: Primer on the Metabolic Bone Diseases and Disorders of Mineral Metabolism. USA; 2018. pp. 12-19. DOI: 10.1002/9781119266594.ch2

[46] Šromová V, Sobola D, Kaspar P. A brief review of bone cell function and importance. Cell. 2023;**12**(21):2576. DOI: 10.3390/cells12212576

Chapter 4

Hereditary Hemorrhagic Telangiectasia (HHT)/Osler-Weber-Rendu Syndrome: A Review on Contemporary Knowledge, Its Accompanying Clinical Manifestations, Diagnostics, and Oro-Dental Management Plan

Ziyad S. Haidar

Abstract

HHT/OWRS is a *very* rare, hereditary, genetic autosomal-dominant disorder characterized by local angiodysplasias on skin and mucosae, even more rarely reported in the oral and dental health-related literature. It affects blood vessel formation throughout the body and is often accompanied with recurrent and severe episodes of epistaxis and telangiectasia on the skin and mucous membranes, including oral mucosae; and henceforth, perhaps the first sign of OWRS/HHT that can be initially diagnosed is by us, dentists/odontologists, oral and cranio-maxillo-facial surgeons, and specialized oral, dental, head, face and neck health care providers. Such symptoms may be associated with an IgA deficiency and, rarely, with von Willebrand disease. Thus, we are in an optimal position to detect the OWRS/HHT symptoms early, even if symptoms of other conditions may or do mimic OWRS/HHT oral lesions. Herein, this chapter re-visits and reviews, for the interested clinician, surgeon, scientist, researcher, and *Innovation in Osteogenesis Research* reader, the current knowledge on a very rare yet complex disease. Hence, the aim herein is for it to serve as a reminder as well as a contemporary clinical and surgical guide aiding in detecting, diagnosing, understanding, and efficaciously managing (including *Health Care Information Management*) patients suffering from OWRS or HHT.

Keywords: Osler-Weber-Rendu syndrome, arterio-venous, malformation, epistaxis, hereditary hemorrhagic telangiectasia, Morbus-Osler, dental implications, genetics

1. Introduction

The Osler-Weber-Rendu syndrome (OWRS) or Osler-Weber-Rendu disease (OWRD) is also known as Morbus-Osler disease and hereditary hemorrhagic telangiectasia (HHT), these 2 (or 3) terms (OWRS, OWRD, and HHT) being interchangeably used in oral communications, books/atlases, and scientific publications. "Hereditary" tackles the inherited character of the disease, and the term "hemorrhagic" derived from the Greek "haima" (blood) and "rhegnynai" (flow) describes nosebleeds, blood coughing, and gastrointestinal bleeding. "Telangiectasia," derived from the Greek "telos" (far), "angeion" (vessel), and "ektasis" (expansion), all these together mean or refer to the pathological expansion of the smallest blood vessels (capillaries). In 1864, Henry Gawen Sutton first described HHT, and in 1896, OWRS was readdressed by French physician Henri Jules Louis Marie Rendu [1] who distinguished it from hemophilia. In 1901, it was revisited by Canadian physician Sir William Osler [2], hence the "Osler's Disease," and in 1907, English dermatologist Frederick Parkes Weber continued the characterization of this disease [3]. At last, in 1909, Hanes named this syndrome as "hereditary hemorrhagic telangiectasia," an autosomal dominant trait [3–5], a disorder in which capillaries throughout the body are weakened (vascular dysplasia) in skin and mucosa. This weakness seemingly is due to defective endothelial interconnections [6] where it affects the blood vessels and is characterized by wide-spread telangiectasias that can involve the skin (face, fingers, and occasionally the palms), mucous membranes (oral, nasal, and gastrointestinal), lungs, and brain. Characteristically, telangiectasias do not become apparent before the upper 30s or 40s as they rarely manifest during childhood or adolescence, and once they manifest, expansion in number and area covered occurs and may bleed after minor trauma, or even spontaneously [6], a tendency to bleed. Telangiectasia on skin, oral and perioral tissues, nasal, gastro-intestinal, or urogenital mucosae often leads to bleeding resulting in iron-deficiency anemia, or, rarely, even cardiac failure. Telangiectasia may be observed in any part of the oral cavity and may be particularly conspicuous on the lips [7], as is depicted in the clinical case in **Figure 1**.

OWRS, seemingly, is due to defective endothelial interconnections. Herein, the genetic defect involves endothelial cells that are obviously unable to produce overlapping cytoplasmic villi that normally interdigitate with an adjacent endothelial cell, and this results in an ultrastructural gap between the endothelial cells. The capillaries then spread and balloon into telangiectasias after years of systemic vascular pressure [8]. OWRS is specifically characterized by alterations in the growth factor receptors of blood vessels endothelial; the first detectable pathology is the focal dilation of postcapillary veinules [6–9]. As the lesion begins to enlarge, over time, capillaries have a tendency to completely disappear and produce a complete arteriole and venule connection. The junction between the vein and artery is thin, leading to a dilation in the vessel wall, and this is called or termed "telangiectasia." In a fully developed telangiectasia, the arteriole and/or venule becomes extremely dilated and manifests superficially on skin or mucosal surfaces as a red or purplish dot. Larger vessel dilations, such as those observed in some internal organs, are named arteriovenous malformations or AVMs. Telangiectasias and AVMs are firstly asymptomatic yet have the tendency to rupture, leading to bleeding episodes that can have serious sequels depending on anatomical location, especially in the case of AVMs, as reported by Sharath Kumar and Shapiro [9]. In about 80% of OWRS patients, a family history is realized [6–9]. The disease may be present in childhood and is more often to appear during puberty, but usually manifests during the second and/or third decades of life and is usually fully blown after the age of 35 and becomes progressively worse with increasing age [6, 9]. Briefly, HHT is classified into four types, though more types may exist: HHT types I and II (account for approximately 85% of cases); HHT type III;

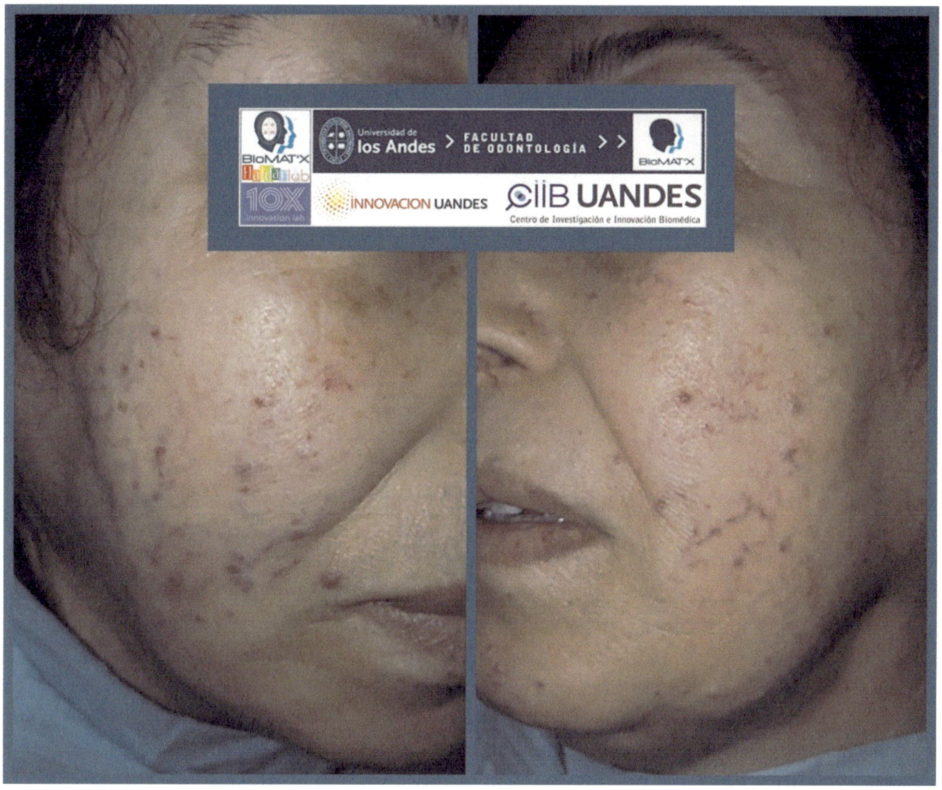

Figure 1.
A 55-year-old woman with OWRS presenting with facial telangiactasis (skin of cheeks and base of nasal pyramid).

and HHT-juvenile polyposis overlap syndrome (JPS-HHT). The juvenile polyposis syndrome (JPS) is a rare autosomal dominant condition (increases the risk of development of gastro-intestinal malignancy) characterized by five or more gastrointestinal tract hamartomatous polyps or one or more juvenile polyps with a family history of JPS [10, 11]. It is worth noting that a juvenile polyposis-hereditary hemorrhagic telangiectasia overlap syndrome has previously been reported in 22% of patients with JPS due to a SMAD4 gene mutation [10–12] or BMPR1A gene, which is found in 40–60% of patients with JPS [11]. In 2012, O'Malley and associates studied and determined the prevalence and clinical manifestations of HHT in their juvenile polyposis patients and concluded that nearly all have the overlap syndrome and that healthcare providers must be aware and cognizant of the juvenile polyposis-hemorrhagic hereditary telangiectasia overlap syndrome [10]. In 2021, the first case of JPS-HHT in South Korea was reported (a 15-year-old boy), exhibiting the performed genetic studies of the patient himself and his parents revealing the detection of a de novo variant in the SMAD4 gene, [SMAD4 c.1146_1163del; p. His382_Val387del] [12]. This report recommended that JPS patients should undergo genetic evaluation of associated genes, including SMAD4, and those patients who are genetically confirmed with SMAD4 variants ought to undergo the appropriate evaluation to detect coexisting asymptomatic AVMs and avert life-threatening complication(s) [12].

2. Epidemiology, etiology, and genetics (+ involved mutations) for HHT type I and II

Given its rarity and scarcity in clinical case reports, no reliable data about the incidence of ORWS exists; the overall prevalence is 1–2 cases per 100,000 in the general North American population according to Marx and Stern [6] and 1 in 5000 to 8000, according to and Begbie et al. [13] and Bailly et al. [14], an underestimation because many cases are asymptomatic (and variable penetrance because main symptoms do not present/appear until later in adult life, in general). Sekarski and Spangenberg [15] and the HHT Foundation International (established in June of 1991 and renamed cure HHT in 2014), reports that more than 1 million cases worldwide are affected by this disorder. OWRS affects men and women in almost equal numbers and manifestations (epistaxis and skin telangiectasias being the most common). Whites are much more frequently affected with HHT than blacks and skin lesions are more common on the face and fingers and are usually well apparent [6]. Children and adults share the same manifestations and parents, once diagnosed, often seek medical attention for their children, with potentially life-threatening manifestations and complications of HHT/OWRS identified in asymptomatic children under 12 years of age [15], rendering screening to recognize this disease (appropriate diagnostic screening), and becoming familiar with evaluation, its manifestations, and treatment options (including prevention of internal bleeding or even death), critical, for the healthcare provider. According to Macri et al. [16] two main types of HHT, HHT1 and HHT2 caused by heterozygous/heterogenic mutations, have been identified, thus far (as of 2022). Briefly, HHT1 involves a mutation (61%) in the ENG gene (endoglin, in chromosome 9, 9q33–34), wherein patients, especially women, are at a higher risk of developing pulmonary and cerebral AVMs. On the other hand, the HHT2 type involves a mutation (37%) in ACVRL1 (activin A receptor-like type 1, in chromosome 12, 12q13) also known as ALK1. Herein, patients tend to have a higher risk of developing AVMs in the liver. Furthermore, mutations in GDF2 (growth differentiation factor 2) that encode the protein that binds to ENG and ACVRL1 have been detected. Both ALK-1 and ENG encode putative receptors for the transforming growth factor-ß (TGF-ß) super-family that plays a crucial role in blood vessels proper development. OWRs, therefore, it has been stated, for decades, to be caused by genetic mutations involving the signaling of TGF-ß, with defects in at least four genes implicated (ENG, ALK1, mutations of chromosome 5, and mutations of SMAD4/MADH4). Mutations in SMAD4/MADH4 (encoding SMAD4 also involves chromosome 18). Today, OWRS/HHT is considered as a disease of the BMP9/10 pathway rather than a disease of the TGF-ß pathway. Furthermore, in dystonia (involuntary muscle contractions) and posture research, genetic studies explained which deletions in 9q34.11 [17] involve the genes ENG, TOR1A (early-onset primary dystonia), STXBP1 (syntaxin binding protein 1 - encephalopathy) and SPTAN 1 (spectrin alpha) are responsible for the multisystemic vascular dysplasia, early-onset dystonia, epilepsy and the intellectual impairment or disability (neuro-developmental disorders/developmental delay), which shows the potential association between dystonia, ±muscle tone, movement disorders, and OWRS.

3. Clinical presentation of OWRS/HHT and its ORO-facial manifestations

OWRS is characterized by spontaneous and recurrent epistaxis, telangiectasia in predetermined areas (oral cavity, nose, fingers, and lips; **Figure 2**), visceral injuries (gastrointestinal, hepatic, pulmonary, cerebral, and spinal), and a family history of HHT. OWRS

DOI: http://dx.doi.org/10.5772/intechopen.1005632

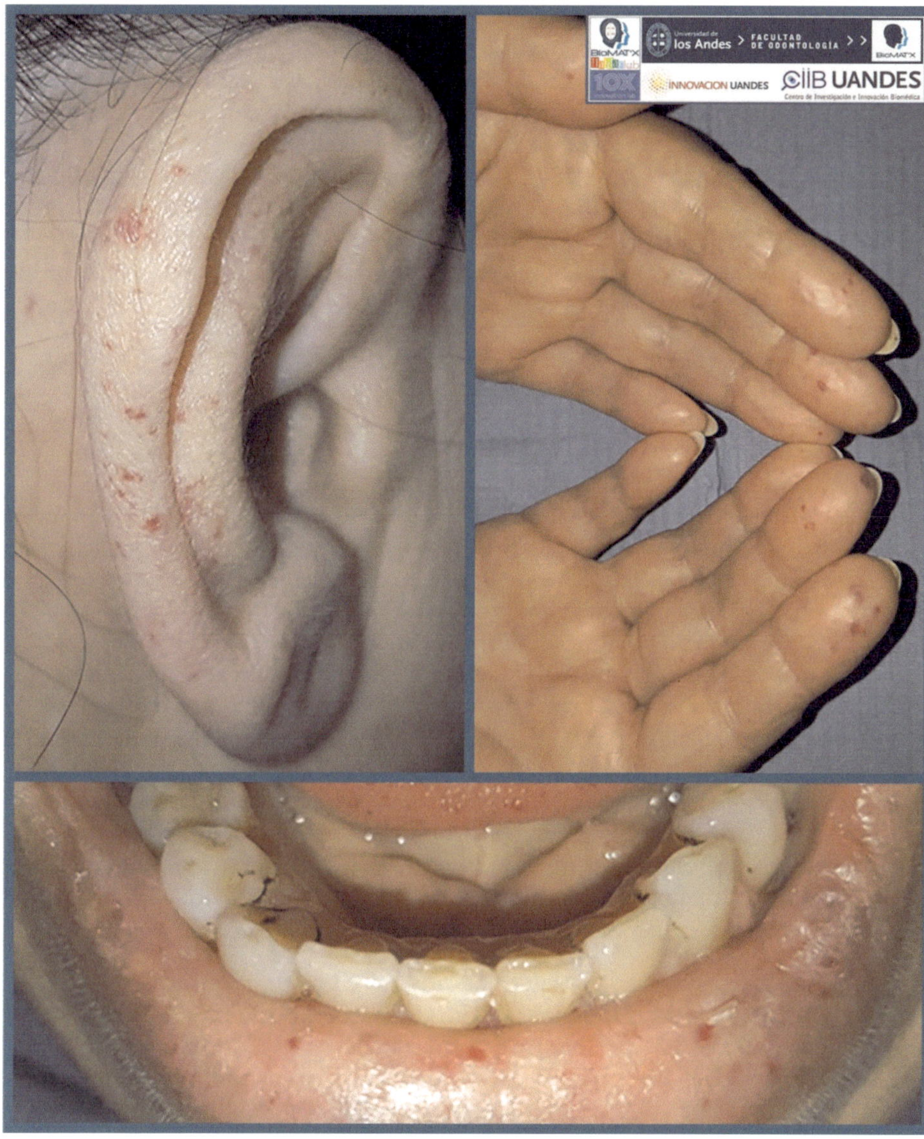

Figure 2.
Same patient in **Figure 1** *with telangiectasias of right external ear, right and left fingertips, and lower lip.*

is an under-diagnosed condition, and without accurate diagnosis, it may lead to serious morbidity and mortality. Clinically, patients develop telangiectatic capillary dilations within the superficial layers of skin and mucous membrane, which always blanch on compression [6, 18, 19]. Below, the most common symptoms and clinical presentation of OWRS/HHT manifestations are summarized to the healthcare attendant:

1. The earliest and most common symptom of OWRS is persistent and recurrent epistaxis (nosebleeds), from childhood. Epistaxis is the most troublesome and most frequently presenting symptom of this multisystem disorder; it is present in more than 90% of affected individuals [20]. It is frequently severe, leading to severe anemia that often necessitates repetitive blood transfusions. On clinical

examination, mucosa of the nasal septum displays small vascular dilations, and epistaxis results from lesions in the anterior septal mucosa within the Kiesselbach's plexus or area (i.e., the wall separating the right and left sides of the nose; a vascular network formed by the five arteries—anastomose—that supply oxygenated blood to the nasal septum, named after the German otolaryngologist Wilhelm Kiesselbach ~ year 1884). It is noteworthy, nonetheless, that while epistaxis in OWRS/HHT can be present all over the nasal surface (medial, lateral, and first 2/3 of the nose), it should not be confused with other unrelated bleedings that can also occur in the *K* area. Such bleedings are often referred to as "*idiopathic hemorrhages*" or "*idiopathic epistaxis.*"

2. Mucocutaneous telangiectasias and angiomas are not generally observed until young adulthood, as tiny red, pulsating, usually punctate, macules and papules (1–3 mm in size) characteristically observed on mucosae and skin, and as skin lesions on trunk and arms, yet more common on the face (base of the nasal pyramid, cheeks, conjunctivae, and ears), and acrally (on peripheral portions of limbs, fingers and toes and nail beds, and head, ears, and nose). These lesions are often red or brown, rather than purple, then readily blanch on diascopy (blanch upon pressure and regain their color when pressure is released). They easily bleed, even after a mild trauma; bleeding is not the result of a deficiency in clotting factor(s), but rather occurs as a result of the rupture of weak capillaries. As the affected patient grows, bleeding episodes increase in intensity and frequency. These diagnostic lesions are also observed within the nasopharynx, gastrointestinal and genitourinary tracts. Note that telangiectasias are permanent small dilations of blood vessels [6] and not angiomas or areas of bleeding; they do not appear characteristically apparent until upper 30s or 40s of age, with rare exceptions manifesting earlier in life. Telangiectasias of the skin and oral mucosae are observed in approximately 75% of patients with OWRS; they are usually visible by age 30,and increase in number and size with age [13]. As mentioned earlier above, the skin lesions occur primarily on the hands, face, and feet [9].

3. GI severe bleeding is also prevalent because of GI telangiectasis. GI bleeding usually recurs in older patients [21]. Gastric, visceral, and lung mucosae may all be involved in OWRS, and because of that, hematemesis (vomiting of blood—indicating upper GI tract bleeding), melena (dark black and tarry feces), or hemoptysis (spitting and coughing of blood originating in the lungs) may be part of the existing symptoms.

4. Visceral arteriovenous malformations or AVMs are also an important manifestation of OWRS, as described earlier. AVMs are observed in different anatomic locations of the body (nasopharynx, central nervous system, lungs, liver, spleen, and, sometimes, on the fingers and tips). Pulmonary, brain, and hepatic AVMs can cause serious complications. Liver lesions occur very frequently in women but the greatest documented risk results from pulmonary areteriovenous fistulae that often predispose patients to septic brain emboli (often lethal), and other central nervous system signs (such as strokes, migraines, and epilepsy) may occur. Cerebral AVMs may lead to headaches, ischemia, seizures, or devastating hemorrhages. Mucocutaneous telangiectasias (occur in about 75% of patients with the condition and are most common to be present on the lips, tongue, buccal mucosa, and fingertips) and AVMs (+ brain/cerebral) are a potential source of serious morbidity and mortality.

5. As consequence of chronic low-level blood loss, iron-deficiency anemia may develop—a condition in which the blood lacks sufficient healthy red blood cells. Without enough iron, the body cannot produce enough hemoglobin in the red blood cells that enable them to carry oxygen. As a result, iron-deficiency anemia may leave the patient feeling tired/fatigued, chest pains, and shortness of breath. Other signs and symptoms may include weakness, headache, dizziness, cold hands and feet, pale skin, brittle nails, poor appetite, and sometimes unusual cravings for nonnutritive substances (starch, ice, or dirt) and inflammation and soreness of the tongue.

6. Spleen and liver vascular anomalies may also occur and are usually associated with liver cirrhosis (scar tissue replaces the healthy tissue) and parenchymal proliferations.

7. In rare cases, some blood coagulation and clotting abnormalities (such as von Willebrand disease or vWD, low level of vWD factor) may be associated with OWRS.

8. For the oral and cranio-maxillo-facial surgeon, OWRS has also been associated with FCOD [22] or florid cemento-osseous dysplasia (a benign fibro-osseous lesion, characterized by the replacement of normal bone with fibrous tissue and metaplastic/nonneoplastic bone in the periapical region of the tooth-bearing jaw areas, predominantly in the mandible, suggested to originate from the periodontal ligament).

Technical note: Given the wide variability in disease expression and severity, in addition to OWRS/HHT established to affect multiple organ systems, several scaling and grading tools have been developed and validated over the years. Indeed, ESS or the epistaxis severity score, the HHT-score, and the Bergler-Sadick scale, among other instruments and PROM or patient-reported outcome measures (such as daily diaries), are available (*classification criteria can vary though Food and Drug Administration or FDA guidance criteria for weighing PROM instruments exist*) to aid in (a) measuring the frequency and intensity of epistaxis and (b) rank disease severity, to properly assess the specific or individual case of OWRS/HHT and OWRS/HHT-related epistaxis. For example, the Bergler-Sadick criteria to scale the severity of epistaxis or nose-bleeds in OWRS/HHT patients go as follows: *GRADE I* (Frequency: ≤ Once a Week; Quantity: Stains on Napkin); *GRADE II* (Frequency: Several per Week; Quantity: Soaked Napkin); and *GRADE III* (Frequency: Daily or Several per Week; Quantity: Bowl or similar utensil deemed necessary). Henceforth, several scales do take into consideration the impact of the disease and its symptoms on quality of life. For instance, besides frequency and quantity of epistaxis, the ESS considers the characteristics of bleeding, presence of anemia, and hospital requirements in addition to the general QoL impact secondary to associated symptoms.

3.1 Orofacial manifestations

In OWRS/HHT, lesions in the oral cavity (**Figure 3**) are most remarkable and noteworthy on the mucosae of dorsal tongue, palate, lips, and buccal mucosa; however, remember, any type of oral mucosa can be affected [23, 24]. Herein, the intraoral lesions are either macular (flat) or papular (elevated), and they usually

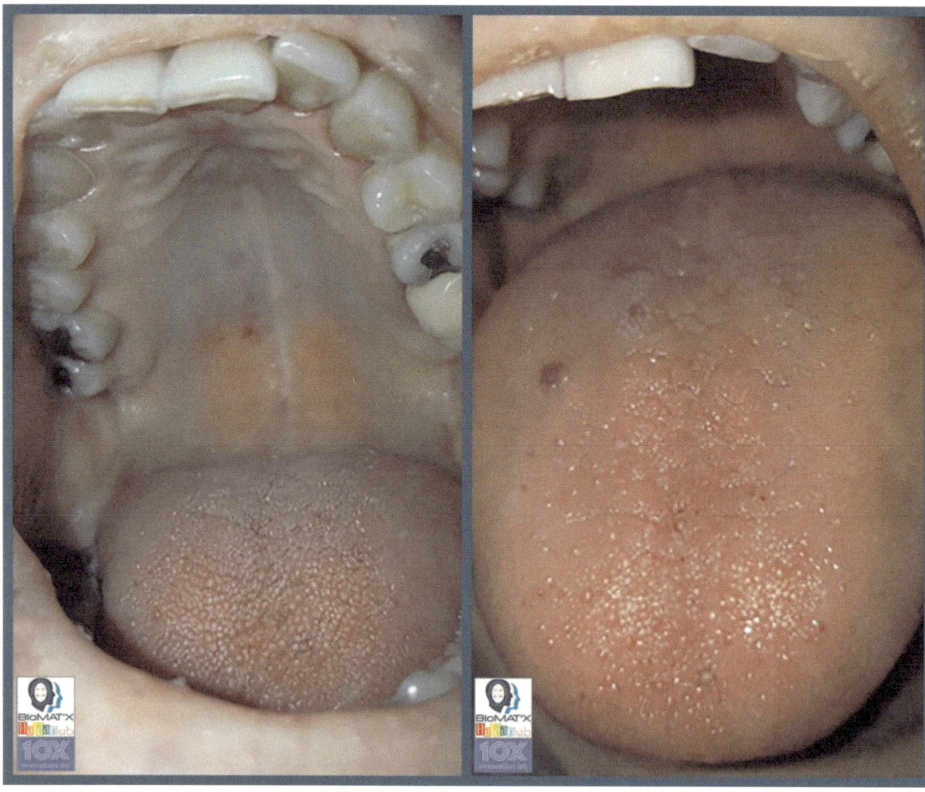

Figure 3.
Telangiectasias on palate and dorsal tongue in the same patient as in the previous figures.

present as "pinpoint-sized" or "pea-sized," and less commonly, may be linear in appearance. With their red/purple appearance, they may resemble mucocutaneous petechiae, yet, unlike petechiae, OWRS telangiectasias blanch upon applying pressure (diascopy test). They are asymptomatic but have a tendency to rupture, leading to oral bleedings. Tens (sometimes hundreds) of round or oval macules/papules are observed on the perioral soft tissues (mucosal base of the nasal pyramid) and inside the oral cavity, particularly on the dorsal tongue and mucosal surface of the lips (vermilion zone), and less often, on the gingiva, palatal mucosa, and buccal mucosa [14, 18, 23, 24]. Lips and tongue are characteristically the prime areas for small pinpoint-sized telangiectasias. Mucocutaneous telangiectasias are observed in about 90% of OWRS cases [25, 26]. and histopathologically are displayed as a superficial collection of dilated blood vessels with a lamina propria characterized by a layer of endothelial cells. The most frequent and worrisome clinical symptom is epistaxis (nosebleed recurrent epistaxis in both children and adults.), as mentioned earlier, from lesions located in the Kiesselbach's plexus (**Figure 4**), which lies within the Kiesselbach's triangle (also known as Little's area in some resources), an anatomical region located in the anteroinferior part of the nasal septum where four (or five) arteries anastomose to form a very rich vascular plexus; these arteries are the anterior ethmoidal artery (branch of ophthalmic artery), the greater palatine artery (branch of maxillary artery), the septal branch of superior labial artery (branch of facial artery), and the sphenopalatine artery (terminal branch of maxillary artery). It is important to notice that 90% of nosebleeds occur in Little's area as this area is constantly exposed to

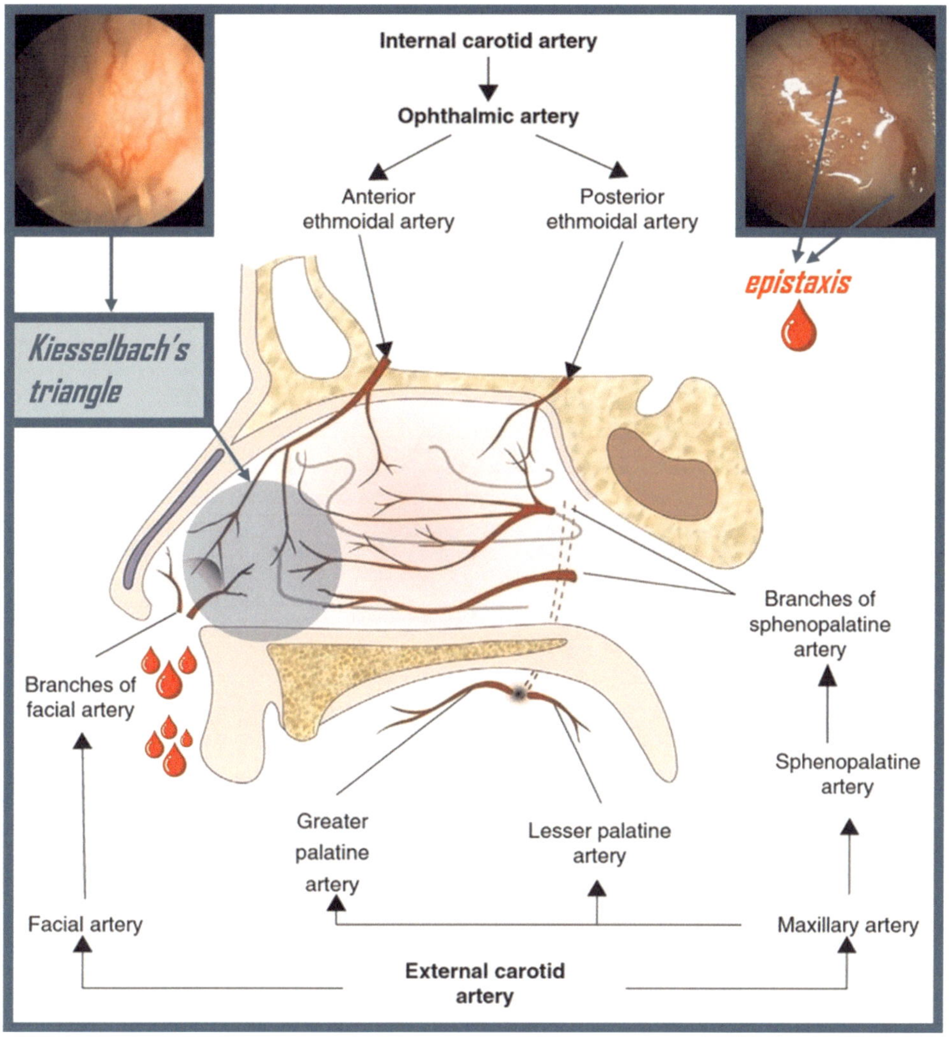

Figure 4.
Epistaxis and the Kiesselbach plexus (triangle or area) supplying blood to the anterioro-inferior quadrant of the nasal septum.

fingernail trauma and to the drying effect of inspiratory currents. Blood in this area is then drained by the facial vein, ophthalmic veins, and the pterygoid plexus. It is noteworthy to mention herein that it is exceptionally rare for a single patient to present with all the "outlined" clinical manifestations of OWRS. It is also noteworthy, as previously mentioned, that while epistaxis in OWRS/HHT can be present over the oral and nasal mucosal surfaces, it should not be clinically confused with other unrelated or idiopathic hemorrhages/epistaxis that can ensue in the *K*-area.

3.2 Diagnosis (D_x)

D_x— Today, OWRS/HHT clinical diagnosis [20] remains based on the "Curaçao Criteria," established in 1999 by the Scientific Advisory Board of the HHT Foundation

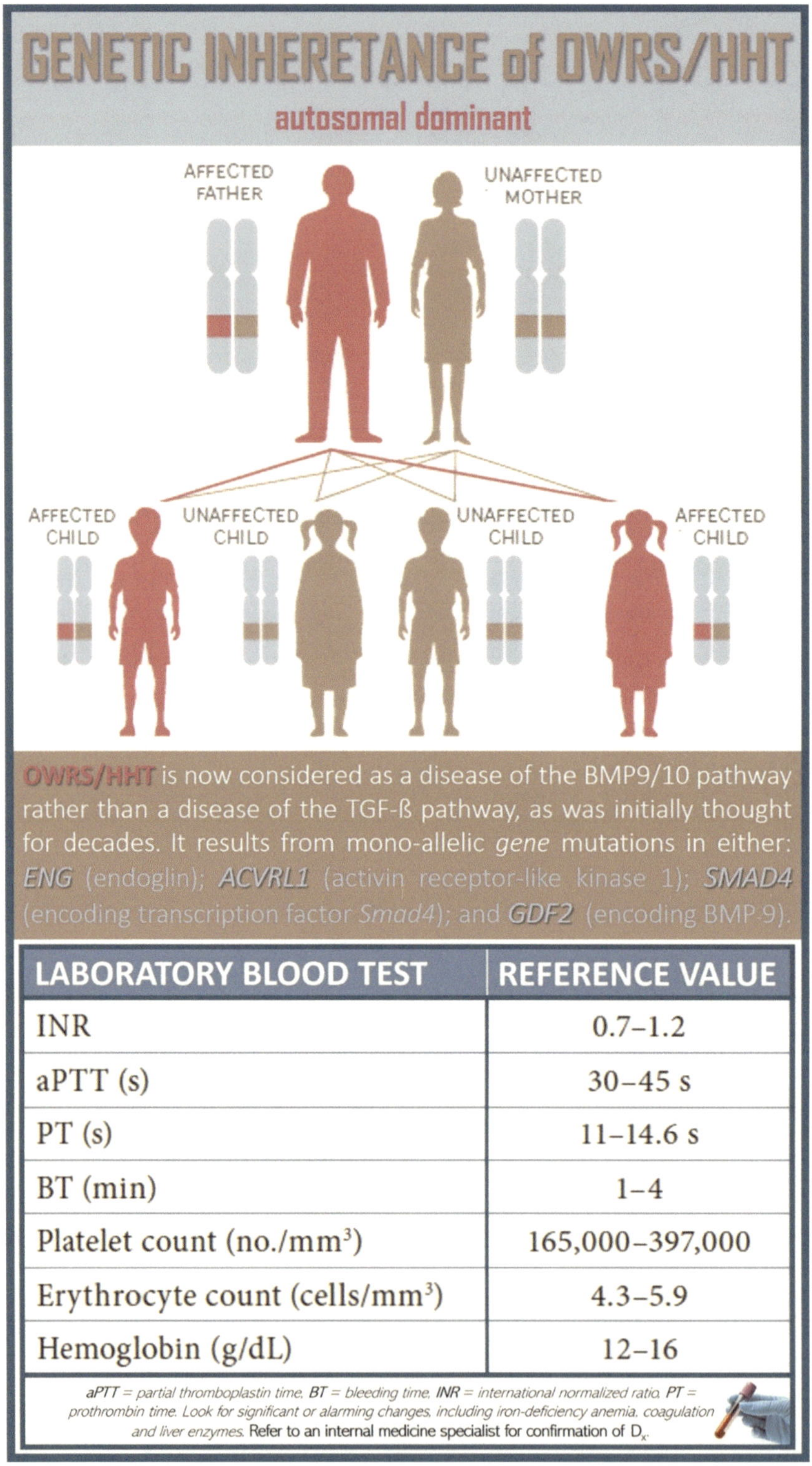

OWRS/HHT is now considered as a disease of the BMP9/10 pathway rather than a disease of the TGF-ß pathway, as was initially thought for decades. It results from mono-allelic *gene* mutations in either: *ENG* (endoglin); *ACVRL1* (activin receptor-like kinase 1); *SMAD4* (encoding transcription factor *Smad4*); and *GDF2* (encoding BMP-9).

LABORATORY BLOOD TEST	REFERENCE VALUE
INR	0.7–1.2
aPTT (s)	30–45 s
PT (s)	11–14.6 s
BT (min)	1–4
Platelet count (no./mm^3)	165,000–397,000
Erythrocyte count (cells/mm^3)	4.3–5.9
Hemoglobin (g/dL)	12–16

aPTT = partial thromboplastin time. BT = bleeding time. INR = international normalized ratio. PT = prothrombin time. Look for significant or alarming changes, including iron-deficiency anemia, coagulation and liver enzymes. Refer to an internal medicine specialist for confirmation of D_x.

Figure 5.
Blood work (CBC: Complete Blood Count) laboratory testing conducted for D_x/DD_x.

DOI: http://dx.doi.org/10.5772/intechopen.1005632

International (Cure HHT in 2014). The four diagnostic criteria of Cure HHT are as follows:

1. Spontaneous and recurrent epistaxis (up to 30 episodes per week). No consensus on number of bleeding episodes or degree of epistaxis necessary for diagnosis; however, nighttime nosebleeds should be considered as especially suspicious;

2. Multiple cutaneous and mucosal telangiectasias in the typical and characteristic locations (tongue, lips, face, extremities of fingers, etc ...) that blanch on diascopy (use a clear glass to press against skin to empty blood from lesion, under pressure);

3. Clinically-proven visceral AVMs (lungs, liver, brain, spine); and Family history in a first-degree relative with OWRS/HHT.

Briefly, if three out of the four criteria are met, the diagnosis of OWRS/HHT is definitive. If only two criteria are present, the diagnosis is considered possible or suspected, and if the patient presents only one criterion, the diagnosis of OWRS/HHT is deemed unlikely. Remember, this is a genetically transmitted disease/condition, and it is inherited as an autosomal dominant trait. As described earlier, genetic testing of patients and their family members can confirm the presence of specific mutations with implicated genes. Herein, it is important to note that some families do not or cannot show a link to any of the known loci. Consequently, children have a 50% chance of contracting this disorder. Screening of family members for signs of OWRS/HHT should include a complete history, physical examination, chest radiography, and arterial blood gas testing (with measurement of the shunt fraction). Recent breakthroughs in molecular genetics have provided the medical community with a deeper understanding of this genetic disorder, but, variability–even among members of the same family renders the D_x tricky. Also, remember that the severity of this genetic disorder largely varies, even between close relatives. Precise testing is advised.

3.3 Differential diagnosis (DDx)

DD_x— Reference to laboratory testing (blood work, **Figure 5**) and an internal medicine specialist is critical, for confirming the D_x agreeing to the Curaçao Criteria. In DD_x, note:

1. In some cases, multiple telangiectasis can be associated with connective tissue disorders, such as the CREST syndrome [26, 27], hence may cause confusion, because of telangiectasia. CREST (Calcinosis, Raynaud's phenomenon, Esophageal dysmotility, Sclerodactyly, Telangiectasia) is the predominantly acral form of PSS or progressive systemic sclerosis (known as scleroderma) in which narrowed lips turn to microstomia and opening the mouth becomes a real problem. CREST syndrome features finger, facial, and oral telangiectasias somehow similar to those of/in OWRS; yet, PSS patients have anti-centromere antibodies, a finding not seen in OWRS/HHT.

2. Fabry syndrome or disease [28] may also manifest with multiple vascular lesions, particularly diffuse full-body telangiectasias that do not blanch upon pressure, as in OWRS/HHT; these telangiectasias and skin lesions begin in childhood and increase (in number and anatomical locations) with age. Fabry syndrome or

Anderson-Fabry disease or angiokeratoma corporis diffusum is a rare genetic (X-linked, passed from parent to child) lysosomal storage disease (typically associated with an enzyme deficiency in the metabolism of glycoprotein, lipids, and fat) that can cause a range of systemic symptoms. This disorder leads to excessive deposition of neutral glycosphingolipids in the vascular endothelium of several organs, and progressive endothelial accumulation of glycosphingolipids will account for associated anomalies of skin, eye (corneal whorls), the peripheral nervous system, kidney, heart, and brain.

3. Mafucci syndrome [29] is a sporadic congenital disease featuring multiple enchondromas (benign enlargements of cartilage) and deformities of metacarpal bones and hand phalanges, multiple cutaneous spindle cell hemangiomas (notably, small tongue hemangiomas) and lymphangiomas, and phleboliths. Enchondromas of the digits are observed in childhood with hands and feet becoming distorted. Etio-pathogenic cause remains unknown, and the risk of sarcomatous (malignant) transformation of enchondromas, hemangiomas, or lymphangiomas is about 15–30%.

4. OWRS should be differentiated from benign hereditary telangiectasis (genetic tests).

5. Cherry angiomas (Campbell de Morgan spots) develop in more than 85–90% of adults over 30–40 years old; these lesions may look similar but are less clustered and more diffuse than of/in OWRS/HHT. Furthermore, those spots or moles [30] do not increase in number with age. Briefly, cherry angiomas are round skin growths that appear bright red in color (hence, “cherry”), and mostly develop on the trunk or torso.

6. Spider nevi (also known as spider telangiectasias, spider angiomas, vascular spider, or nevus araneus) may also mimic OWRS/HHT lesions [31]; they present as a developmental malformation in children and adolescents, as multiple or solitary lesions, and do not change during adult life. These vascular lesions (characterized by anomalous dilatation of end vasculature) are a type of telangiectasis found beneath the skin surface. These lesions, typically painless, can be observed anywhere on the body, most common on the face, neck, and legs (sun-exposed areas). However, having more than three spider angiomas is likely to be an abnormality and is a physically- diagnostic sign of liver disease in adults (seen in many alcoholics with liver cirrhosis).

3.4 Diagnostic workup and progrnosis

Diagnostic work-up— Recurrent and persistent severe bleeding episodes may lead to an iron-deficiency anemia [26], as mentioned earlier, requiring regular blood work (CBC: Complete blood count) with an assessment of Wintrobe indices (hematocrit, MCV, MCH, MCHC) in order to measure quantitatively the red blood cell population, serum iron, and the total iron binding capacity. In the case of a gastrointestinal bleeding, a gastroscopy and a colonoscopy may be indicated by the attending physician. AVMs are obviously the most dangerous complication of OWRS/HHT; approximately, 30% of patients will develop pulmonary AVMs, which usually develop during puberty, and 10% will develop cerebral AVMs (which may be lethal). Screening for

DOI: http://dx.doi.org/10.5772/intechopen.1005632

OWRS should also include a contrast echocardiography of the lungs and magnetic resonance imaging/MRI of the brain. After confirming the diagnosis, angiography and magnetic resonance angiogram/MRA scans are to be done in order to assess the AVMs. Genetic counseling is strongly advised, and genetic testing is favored in families with history of OWRS/HHT.

Prognosis of OWRS/HHT— relatively good although morbidity is significant. Life expectancy may be shortened; however, this depends on the severity of symptoms and the manifestations/complications of the disease, and the degree of systemic involvement (especially hepatic, pulmonary, and central nervous system involvement). Briefly, mortality shows an early peak at the age of 50 years and a later peak at 60–80 years, this being related to acute complications [19, 20, 27]. Only, 10% of patients die of complications. Patients with AVMs may experience early-onset stroke and brain abscesses, and it is estimated that a mortality rate of 1–2% is due to complications related to epistaxis, and it rises to 10% in patients with cerebral abscesses [32]. In general, the disease prognosis remains good and acceptable as long as the bleeding episodes are promptly identified and adequately controlled. OWRS/HHT is often unrecognized by physicians and other health care providers, as emphasized earlier. In 2012, the HHT Foundation estimated that 9 out of 10 people with OWRS go undiagnosed, and among individuals with un-diagnosed OWRS, 20% are either disabled or die because healthcare providers failed to recognize and subsequently treat or manage the disease. If properly diagnosed, AVMs and complications can be prevented.

3.5 Management and Rx

Management and R_x— OWRS/HHT are obviously not curable, yet, are manageable. Nowadays, it is worldwide accepted that no treatment is indicated other than local hemostatic measures during the bleeding episodes. Currently-used “therapeutic” protocols are essentially symptomatic, dealing with symptoms and signs rather than the disease itself and knowing that no therapy is able to stop the development of AVMs and telangiectasias. The following “therapeutic” modalities, deduced from various resources, clinical case studies, and series, might be perhaps useful in the management of OWRS:

1. Spontaneous bleedings are controlled by pressure packs (Ethicon surgical dressing, for example), and particularly nasal bleedings. Packing of the nasal cavity with absorbent swabs or gels is a very popular method and LASER coagulation therapy [33] also works relatively well for nasal telangiectasias that cause the nosebleeds.

2. Silver-nitrate (chemical cautery), electric cautery (hotwire or bipolar cautery), and Nd: YAG laser pulse dye laser [34], or combinations of those techniques, are prophylactically used by some clinicians in lesions that are more likely to bleed and for the destruction of cutaneous and accessible mucosal lesions. Nasal coagulation and cauterization may reduce bleeding (once the bleeding point is identified) resulting from telangiectasias and is currently recommended before surgery is indicated (often, several cauterization/coagulation sessions are needed).

3. If all interventions to stop epistaxis have failed, special procedures have to be considered, such as septal dermoplasty, also known as Saunder’s procedure

[35], in which skin is transplanted into the nostrils in order to replace the involved mucosae and Young's procedure [36] in which nostrils are completely sealed off.

4. Corticosteroid nasal sprays, such as beclomethasone dipropionate (inhaled form is used in the management of asthma), often reduce minor recurrent nasal bleeds.

5. Sclerosing agents (such as sodium morrhuate and sodium tetradecyl sulfate) can be injected into OWRS/HHT lesions.

6. Lung lesions are currently managed by transcatheter embolization (blocking off the feeding artery). Brain AVMs are managed with more than one modality (surgical removal, embolization, or treating the affected area with radiation), depending on location, size, and structure of the abnormal vessels.

7. Chronic and repeated epistaxis and GI bleedings often lead to severe anemia, requiring iron supplements. Patients who cannot tolerate iron solutions or tablets usually require administration of IV iron sucrose and blood transfusions if the anemia causes severe symptoms that urgently warrant rapid recovery of the CBC.

8. Other therapies, such as estrogen-containing creams, progesterone, and oral tranexamic acid, were also suggested in the medical literature.

4. Dental aspects and implications of HHT

After epistaxis, oral bleeding is the second most frequent and annoying complaint of ORWS/HHT patients. Though relatively uncommon, oral bleeding may be the result of traumatic tooth brushing or after an inadvertent bite of the oral soft tissues or following an oral surgical procedure [37–41]. In everyday general dental practice, gingival bleeding upon oral debridement (scaling/root planning) and post-extraction hemorrhage are a prime concern for dentists. Herein, drugs, such as aspirin and non-steroidal anti-inflammatory drugs (diclofenac, ibuprofen, naproxen, etc…) should be strictly avoided due to the elevated risk of bleeding [15]. In very rare cases, a fatal hemorrhage can happen after a dental or oral surgical procedure [37–44]. Regarding the need for antibiotic prophylaxis before routine dental and oral surgeries (implant placement, surgical extractions, biopsies, cysts, and tumors excision among others,) there is no consensus yet, and to the best of our knowledge and expertise, some patients with OWRS/HHT can develop brain and pulmonary abscesses following teeth extractions in the absence of antibiotic prophylaxis [42–45]. These specific cases confirm the importance of prevention of cerebral and pulmonary abscess with antibiotics in this specific group of patients, despite the absence of evidence of the indication to use antibiotic prophylaxis for OWRS/HHT in the scientific and clinical literature [46]. According to several studies [9, 20], many patients with OWRS/HHT need/require antibiotic prophylaxis before undergoing any dental/oral invasive procedure that may produce a bacteremia (oral debridement, extractions, biopsies, cyst enucleation, implant placement, etc…), and this issue is primarily due to problems resulting from pulmonary AVMs, which obviously lack the capillaries to filter the blood when passing through the lungs, thereby, allowing bacteria to travel to the brain. Indeed, vascular malformations and arteriovenous fistulae in the lungs play an important role in the pathogenesis of a cerebral abscess, and it is known that a peripheral septic microembolism is able to reach the brain and cause a brain abscess [42]. Nowadays, the use of antibiotic prophylaxis preventively remains empirical for OWRS/HHT dental patients; nonetheless, most dental clinicians prefer to implement protocols before dental/oral invasive procedures in order to avoid the development of a cerebral abscess. If a patient with OWRS/HHT was not tested properly to have the diagnostics for AVMs, dental treatment should be mandatorily delayed until appropriate testing is done and completed [23, 42, 47]. Medication before dental/oral invasive procedures is not necessary for OWRS patients who present with AVMs in other organs but is mandatory for those with pulmonary AVMs that occur in approximately a third of OWRS patients and may lead to many complications. Among those, pulmonary hemorrhage, cerebral embolism, and hypoxia have been reported [48, 49]. Consequently, dentists must keep the dental chair in a vertical position during the treatment sessions and be prepared, at any time, to administer oxygen [42]. OWRS/HHT patients with severe anemia (hemoglobin level less than 10 mg/dL) better avoid such invasive procedures as well as might exacerbate anemia, depending on the lost amount of blood [50]. Regional analgesia of nerve trunks (such as the inferior alveolar nerve) also should be better avoided due to the risk of bleeding (nerve accidental trauma with the anesthetic needle), and, for the general anesthesia of dental patients, nasal intubation is better be avoided.

Pharmaceutical note: As described earlier, epistaxis due to rupture of telangiectases of the nasal mucosa is the most frequent clinical manifestation in OWRS/HHT patients. Epistaxis leads, in many cases, to severe impairment of QoL, which is also known to worsen with age, among other physiological, psycho-socio-economic factors and lifestyle parameters. Daiana de Morais and group [51–54] investigated and reported on more than 15 years of using several sub-mucosal or sub-pericondrial treatments aimed at reducing epistaxis in OWRS/HHT patients. They have concluded that sub-mucosal 1–2 mL injections of 0.5% polidocanol, also known as lauromacrogol 400 (Aethoxysklerol®, Kreussler Pharma, Ferrer Farma S.A, Spain), improved nosebleeds (in frequency and quantity) in 95% of all the cases studied (N=45 patients diagnosed with OWRS/HHT based on the clinical Curaçao criteria; ~245–300 infiltrations administered using 25-gauge needles in the septum or in the telangiectasia area, at the ENT/Otorhinolaryngology unit of the Valladolid University Hospital in Valladolid, Spain), without any significant side effects. The authors reported that the average number of sclerosing infiltrations per patient was 5–6 in each nasal cavity. They only administered the polidocanol injections in one nasal cavity and never bilaterally at the same time. Aethoxysklerol® as a sclerosant / anti-angiogenic has a concentration-dependent effect on the endothelium of blood vessels, often used for the treatment of treatment of varicose/spider veins and hemorrhoids. The active sclerosan polidocanol, a solvent and non-ionic emulsifier that contains 95% hydroxypolyethoxydodecane and 5% ethyl alcohol, has been described to form aggregations of molecules (in micellar form), to act as a detergent and has been used as an anaesthetic or an anti-pruritic in medicaments.

In a recent systematic review [55] of a total of 21 randomized controlled clinical trials, the obtained data were pooled for qualitative- and meta-analysis. Treatments included timolol, propranolol, bevacizumab, doxycycline, tacrolimus, estriol/estradiol, tranexamic acid, tamoxifen, sclerosing agent, electrosurgical plasma coagulation, KTP laser, and post-operative packing. Interestingly, propranolol was concluded to offer the most improved epistaxis severity score, when compared to placebo, followed by timolol. The analysis also showed that tranexamic acid significantly reduced the frequency of epistaxis. Briefly, the authors concluded that propranolol, timolol, tranexamic acid, tamoxifen, and estriol were effective for epistaxis management in OWRS/HHT patients. The study also noted the potential post-therapeutic adverse events and impact on QoL Herein, remember that lifestyle and dietary factors do influence the severity of epistaxis. Indeed, while alcohol and salicylates such as red wine, coffee, spices, and chocolate are reported in the literature to exacerbate epistaxis, room humidification and nasal lubrication can help improve the nose-bleeds and the QoL of our OWRS/HHT patients.

5. Key points to note: Contemporary clinical and innovation summary

5.1 Bone-related manifestations

While the primary symptoms of OWRS/HHT typically involve the skin and mucous membranes (nosebleeds, telangiectasias, and arteriovenous malformations), the disorder can also affect other parts of the body, including the bones. Some of the rare (or not so well-documented) and possible bone-related symptoms and manifestations of OWRS/HHT may include Osteoporosis: Osteoporosis is a condition characterized by reduced bone density and increased susceptibility to fractures due to the weakening of bone tissue. OWRS/HHT can cause a decrease in bone mineral density, leading to osteoporosis, which is characterized by weakened bones and an increased risk of fractures. Avascular necrosis: Avascular necrosis is a condition in which bone tissue dies due to a lack of blood supply, leading to bone collapse and joint damage. The abnormal blood vessels in OWRS/HHT can affect blood flow to the bones, potentially leading to avascular necrosis, a condition in which bone tissue dies due to a lack of blood supply. Osteoarthritis: Osteoarthritis is a degenerative joint disease characterized by the breakdown of cartilage and bones in the joints, resulting in pain, stiffness, and loss of function. The abnormal blood vessels and inflammation associated with OWRS/HHT can contribute to the development of osteoarthritis, a degenerative joint disease that affects the cartilage and bones in the joints. Bone abscesses: Bone abscesses are collections of pus within bone tissue, typically caused by bacterial infection and characterized by pain, swelling, and localized inflammation. OWRS/HHT can increase the risk of infections in the bone, leading to the formation of bone abscesses. Pathological fractures: Pathological fractures are fractures that occur in weakened or diseased bone, typically due to underlying conditions, such as osteoporosis or bone cancer. Weakened bones and bone infections associated with OWRS/HHT can increase the risk of pathological fractures, which occur when a bone breaks due to an underlying disease or condition(s).

5.2 Innovations in OWRS/HHT research

There are several innovative approaches being explored to address OWRS/HHT and its bone-related manifestations. While there is currently no cure for OWRS/HHT, advancements in research and treatment options are helping to improve outcomes and quality of life for individuals with the condition. Some of the key innovations in this field include Targeted therapies: Researchers are investigating targeted therapies that aim to block specific molecular pathways involved in OWRS/HHT, such as the vascular endothelial growth factor (VEGF) pathway. Drugs, such as bevacizumab (Avastin) and thalidomide (Thalomid) have shown promise in reducing bleeding and stabilizing telangiectasias in some patients. Gene therapy: Gene therapy is a cutting-edge approach that involves modifying a patient's genetic material to correct a faulty gene or introduce a functional gene. In the case of OWRS/HHT, researchers are exploring the use of gene therapy to target the underlying genetic mutations responsible for the disorder. Angiogenesis inhibitors: Angiogenesis inhibitors are drugs that prevent the formation of new blood vessels. These drugs are being studied for their potential to reduce bleeding and stabilize telangiectasias in patients with OWRS/HHT. Surgical interventions: Surgical interventions, such as embolization or laser therapy, are used to treat severe bleeding or arteriovenous malformations (AVMs) in patients with OWRS/HHT. These procedures aim to block abnormal blood vessels or reduce blood flow to affected areas. Stem cell therapy: Stem cell therapy is an emerging field that holds promise for regenerating damaged tissues and organs. While still in the early stages of research, stem cell therapy may offer potential benefits for individuals with OWRS/HHT and bone-related manifestations by promoting bone repair and regeneration. Biologics: Biologics are a class of drugs derived from living organisms, such as proteins or antibodies. Some biologics have shown promise in reducing inflammation and tissue damage associated with OWRS/HHT and its bone-related manifestations. Patient education and support: In addition to medical treatments, patient education, and support play a crucial role in managing OWRS/HHT and its complications. Support groups and online resources can provide valuable information and support for individuals with OWRS/HHT and their families. Furthermore, it is perhaps noteworthy herein that many of these innovations are still in the early stages of research and may not be widely available. Additionally, the effectiveness of aforementioned treatments can vary from person to person, and more research is needed to fully understand their long-term effects and safety. However, these advancements offer hope for improved outcomes and quality of life for individuals living with OWRS/HHT and its bone-related manifestations. It is also perhaps mentioning that nanotechnology as well can and will contribute to develop novel therapeutic strategies for such bone-related manifestations of OWRS/HHT, offering several potential benefits, not limited to. Drug delivery: Nanoparticles can be engineered to carry drugs or therapeutic agents directly to bone tissue, enabling targeted treatment of bone-related complications, such as osteoporosis or avascular necrosis. Bone regeneration: Nanomaterials can be used to develop scaffolds or matrixes that promote bone growth and repair, addressing bone defects or fractures caused by OWRS/HHT. Imaging: Nanoparticles can be designed to enhance the detection and imaging of bone lesions, allowing for more accurate diagnosis and monitoring of bone-related complications in patients with OWRS/HHT. Theranostics: Nanotechnology can enable the development of theranostic agents that combine therapeutic and diagnostic capabilities, offering a personalized approach to the treatment of bone-related manifestations in OWRS/HHT. Antiangiogenic Therapy: Nanoparticles can be engineered to deliver antiangiogenic agents directly to abnormal blood vessels associated with OWRS/HHT, potentially reducing the risk of bleeding and stabilizing telangiectasias. While nanotechnology holds great promise for addressing various medical conditions, extending to tackling the complex bone-related manifestations of OWRS/HHT by providing targeted and personalized therapeutic options, it is nonetheless important to note that many of these applications are still in the early stages of research, development, and innovation and more studies are needed to fully understand their effectiveness and safety in clinical settings, topics of ongoing investigation at our BioMAT'X I + D + i (HAiDAR R&D&I) Lab at Universidad de los Andes in Santiago de Chile.

6. Conclusions and perspective

OWRS is a multisystem disorder. It is manageable but obviously not curable. The symptoms of OWRS/HHT are often unrecognized; hence, many patients, even those with affected and diagnosed family members, may go un-diagnosed. Clinical diagnosis, typically, is based on the presence of three of four criteria: epistaxis, telangiectasias, visceral arteriovenous malformations, and/or a family history of the disease. Many patients do not need any treatment, and those who need intervention, typically, are those who suffer from regular and severe epistaxis. Most importantly, to limit the morbidity and mortality associated with OWRS/HHT, its manifestations, and complications, some of which can be lethal recommendations for diagnostic screening, monitoring, and proper management of signs and symptoms have been created. Such, if implemented, have contributed to the prognosis (and survival) of OWRS/HHT. This article attempted to provide the health care personnel, attendants, and professionals, particularly those involved in the dental and cranio-maxillo-facial field (as potentially the front liner or first to detect the present vascular changes/malformations intraorally and facially and aid in diagnosis) with a concise yet comprehensive review (and guide) of the condition, its clinical presentation, and management strategies, most of which are palliative. Indeed, medical intervention in OWRS/HHT depends on the severity of its manifestations and stage of the condition and its accompanying complications. Remember, oral lesions, which later become obvious through hemorrhagic telangiectasia, are often the first sign of this disease. Further, TMJ (temporomandibular joint) dislocation has been associated with OWRS/HHT. Also and generally, the disease/condition depends on the age of the patient. To control epistaxis, surgical intervention is becoming routine. Hemostatic cautery (and skin grafting) procedures have been reported as well with good results; specifically, to reduce long-term oral bleeding. The dentist (and dental hygienist) is to be cautious when attending patients with pulmonary and cerebral AVMS given their high risk of developing abscesses from dental bacteremia, post-routine, and/or invasive oral, dental, and periodontal procedures. On the other hand, despite the constantly accruing advances in understanding the underlying signaling and genetic mutation mechanisms (evident by the recent discovery that OWRS/HHT is a disease of the BMP9/10 pathway rather than a disease of the TGF-ß pathway, as was initially thought for decades), the rare OWRS/HHT continues to pose a perplexing challenge to medicine, pathologists, and biologists, rendering the need for more studies and analysis. Yet, on an optimistic closing note, innovative mechanism-driven pharmaceuticals can be someday anticipated to be designed, formulated, characterized, evaluated, optimized, and translated to the clinic.

Acknowledgements

This work was supported by operating grants provided to the HAiDAR I + D + i/R&D&I LAB/BioMAT'X (Laboratorio de Biomateriales, Farmacéuticos y Bioingeniería de Tejidos Cráneo Máxilo-Facial), member of CiiB (Centro de Investigación e Innovación Biomédica), Faculties of Medicine and Dentistry, Universidad de los Andes, Santiago de Chile, through the ANID-NAM (Agencia Nacional de Investigación y Desarrollo, Chile and National Academy of Medicine, NIH, USA) Grant código # NAM21I0022 (2020-2022), CORFO Crea y Valida I + D + i

Grant código # 21CVC2-183649 (2021-2023), CORFO Crea y Valida — Proyecto de I + D + i Colaborativo - Reactívate" Grant código # 22CVC2-218196 (2022-2024), and FONDEF Concurso IDEA de I + D, ANID, Grant código # ID22I10215 (2022-2024). The author acknowledges orofacial pathology clinical insights from Dr. Ziad E. F. Noujeim.

Conflict of interest

None.

Author details

Ziyad S. Haidar[1,2,3,4,5]

1 BioMAT'X I+D+i (HAIDAR R&D&I LAB), Universidad de los Andes, Chile

2 Facultad de Odontología, Universidad de los Andes, Chile

3 Centro de Investigación e Innovación Biomédica (CiiB), Universidad de los Andes, Chile

4 Programa de Doctorado en BioMedicina, Facultad de Medicina, Universidad de los Andes, Chile

5 Programa de Doctorado en Ciencias Odontológicas, Facultad de Odontología, Universidad de los Andes, Chile

*Address all correspondence to: zhaidar@uandes.cl

References

[1] Rendu HJ. Epistaxis répétées chez un sujet porteur de petits angiomes cutanés et muqueux. Gaz Hop Paris. 1896;**135**: 1322-1323

[2] Osler W. On a family form of recurring epistaxis associated with multiple telangiectasis of the skin and mucous membranes. Bulletin of the John Hopkins Hospital. 1901;**12**:333-337

[3] Weber FP. Multiple hereditary developmental angiomata (telangiectases) of the skin and mucous membranes associated with recurring haemorrhages. Lancet. 1907;**2**(4377): 160-162

[4] Bird RM. A family reunion: A study of hereditary hemorrhagic telangiectasis. The New England Journal of Medicine. 1957;**257**:105-112

[5] Flint SR, Keith O, Scully C. Hereditary hemorrhagic telangiectasia: Family study and review. Oral Surgery, Oral Medicine, and Oral Pathology. 1988;**66**:440-444

[6] Marx RE, Stern D. Oral and Maxillofacial Pathology: A Rationale for Diagnosis and Treatment. Hanover Park, IL: Quintessence Pub. Co; 2012

[7] Scully C. Oral Medicine and Pathology at a Glance. Chichester, U.K: Wiley-Blackwell; 2010

[8] Marx RE, Stern D. Oral and Maxillofacial Pathology: A Rationale for Diagnosis and Treatment. Chicago: Quintessence Pub. Co; 2003

[9] Sharathkumar AA, Shapiro A. Hereditary haemorrhagic telangiectasia. Haemophilia. 2008;**14**:1269-1280. DOI: 10.1111/j.1365-2516.2008.01774.x

[10] O'Malley M, LaGuardia L, Kalady MF, Parambil J, Heald B, Eng C, et al. The prevalence of hereditary hemorrhagic telangiectasia in juvenile polyposis syndrome. Diseases of the Colon and Rectum. 2012;**55**(8):886-892. DOI: 10.1097/DCR.0b013e31825aad32

[11] Cohen S, Hyer W, Mas E, Auth M, Attard TM, Spalinger J, et al. Management of juvenile polyposis syndrome in children and adolescents: A position paper from the ESPGHAN polyposis working group. Journal of Pediatric Gastroenterology and Nutrition. 2019;**68**(3):453-462. DOI: 10.1097/MPG.0000000000002246

[12] Kang B, Hwang SK, Choi S, Kim ES, Lee SY, Ki CS, et al. Case report of juvenile polyposis/hereditary hemorrhagic telangiectasia syndrome: First report in Korea with a novel mutation in the SMAD4 gene. Translational Pediatrics. 2021;**10**(5): 1369-1376. DOI: 10.21037/tp-21-12

[13] Begbie ME, Wallace GM, Shovlin CL. Hereditary haemorrhagic telangiectasia (Osler-Weber-Rendu syndrome): A view from the 21st century. Postgraduate Medical Journal. 2003;**79**(927):18-24. DOI: 10.1136/pmj.79.927.18

[14] Bailly S, Dupuis-Girod S, Plauchu H. Maladie de Rendu-Osler: dysfonctionnement de la signalisation TGF-bêta dans les cellules endothéliales [Rendu-Osler disease: clinical and molecular update]. Medical Science (Paris). 2010;**26**(10):855-860. French. DOI: 10.1051/medsci/20102610855

[15] Sekarski LA, Spangenberg LA. Hereditary hemorrhagic telangiectasia:

Children need screening too. Pediatric Nursing. 2011;**37**(4):163-168; quiz 169

[16] Macri A, Wilson AM, Shafaat O, et al. Osler-Weber-Rendu Disease [Internet]. Treasure Island (FL): StatPearls Publishing; 2022. [Updated 2022 May 3]

[17] Campbell IM, Yatsenko SA, Hixson P, Reimschisel T, Thomas M, Wilson W, et al. Novel 9q34.11 gene deletions encompassing combinations of four Mendelian disease genes: STXBP1, SPTAN1, ENG, and TOR1A. Genetics in Medicine. 2012;**14**:868-876

[18] Govani FS, Shovlin CL. Hereditary haemorrhagic telangiectasia: A clinical and scientific review. European Journal of Human Genetics. 2009;**17**(7):860-871

[19] Dupuis-Girod S, Bailly S, Plauchu H. Hereditary hemorrhagic telangiectasia (HHT): From molecular biology to patient care. Journal of Thrombosis and Haemostasis. 2010;**8**(7):1447-1456

[20] Olitsky SE. Hereditary hemorrhagic telangiectasia: Diagnosis and management. American Family Physician. 2010;**82**(7):785-790

[21] Smith CR Jr, Bartholomew LG, Cain JG. Hereditary hemorrhagic telangiectasia and gastrointestinal hemorrhage. Gastroenterology. 1963;**44**:1-6

[22] Fenerty S, Shaw W, Verma R, Syed AB, Kuklani R, Yang J, et al. Florid cemento-osseous dysplasia: Review of an uncommon fibro-osseous lesion of the jaw with important clinical implications. Skeletal Radiology. 2017;**46**(5):581-590. DOI: 10.1007/s00256-017-2590-0. Epub 2017 Feb 13

[23] Edwards PC, McVaney T. External cervical root resorption involving multiple maxillary teeth in a patient with hereditary hemorrhagic telangiectasia. Oral Surgery, Oral Medicine, Oral Pathology, Oral Radiology, and Endodontics. 2005;**100**(5):585-591. DOI: 10.1016/j.tripleo.2005.02.069

[24] Regezi JA, Sciubba JJ, Jordan RCK. Oral Pathology: Clinical Pathologic Correlations. 6th ed. St Louis: Elsevier Saunders; 2011. p. 388

[25] Folz BJ, Lippert BM, Wollstein AC, Tennie J, Happle R, Werner JA. Mucocutaneous telangiectases of the head and neck in individuals with hereditary hemorrhagic telangiectasia—analysis of distribution and symptoms. European Journal of Dermatology. 2004;**14**(6):407-411

[26] Sadick H, Sadick M, Götte K, et al. Hereditary hemorrhagic telangiectasia: An update on clinical manifestations and diagnostic measures. Wiener Klinische Wochenschrift. 2006;**118**:72-80. DOI: 10.1007/s00508-006-0561-x

[27] de Gussem EM, Kroon S, Hosman AE, Kelder JC, Post MC, Snijder RJ, et al. Hereditary hemorrhagic telangiectasia (HHT) and survival: The importance of systematic screening and treatment in HHT centers of excellence. Journal of Clinical Medicine. 2020;**9**(11): 3581. DOI: 10.3390/jcm9113581

[28] Burand AJ Jr, Stucky CL. Fabry disease pain: Patient and preclinical parallels. Pain. 2021;**162**(5):1305-1321. DOI: 10.1097/j.pain.00000000000 02152

[29] Amyere M, Dompmartin A, Wouters V, Enjolras O, Kaitila I, Docquier PL, et al. Common somatic alterations identified in maffucci syndrome by molecular karyotyping. Molecular Syndromology. 2014;**5**(6):

259-267. DOI: 10.1159/000365898. Epub 2014 Aug 26

[30] Jan W, Din TU, A, Chaudhary FMD, Tameez-Ud-Din A, Nawaz F. Hereditary hemorrhagic telangiectasia: A rare cause of anemia. Cureus. 2019;**11**(8):e5349. DOI: 10.7759/cureus.5349

[31] Samant H, Kothadia JP. Spider Angioma. Treasure Island (FL): StatPearls Publishing; 2022. [Updated 2022 May 8]

[32] Neville BW, Damn DD, Allen CM, Bouquot JE. Oral and Maxillofacial Pathology. 2nd ed. Philadelphia: WB Saunders; 2002. pp. 541-593

[33] Fiorella ML, Lillo L, Fiorella R. Diode laser in the treatment of epistaxis in patients with hereditary haemorrhagic telangiectasia. Acta Otorhinolaryngologica Italica. 2012; **32**(3):164-169

[34] Zhang J. Joint laser photocoagulation and bipolar electrocautery in treating epistaxis. World Journal of Surgery and Surgical Research. 2022;**5**:1373

[35] Saunders WH. Septal dermoplasty: A new operative procedure for control of nosebleeds in patients with hereditary haemorrhagic telangiectasia. The Journal of Laryngology and Otology. 1963;**77**: 69-76

[36] Young A. Closure of the nostrils in allergic rhinitis. The Journal of Laryngology and Otology. 1967;**81**(5): 515-524

[37] Peluse S. Gingival hemorrhage with oral manifestations in hereditary hemorrhagic telangiectasia. Archives of Otolaryngology. 1946;**44**:668-672

[38] Everett FG, Hahn CR. Hereditary hemorrhagic telangiectasiawith gingival lesions: Review and case reports. Journal of Periodontology. 1976;**47**:295-298

[39] Hattler AB, Summers RB. Hereditary hemorrhagic telangiectasia: Report of case and clinical considerations. Journal of the American Dental Association (1939). 1981;**103**:421-422

[40] Austin GB, Quart AM, Novak B. Hereditary hemorrhagic telangiectasia with oral manifestations. Oral Surgery, Oral Medicine, and Oral Pathology. 1981; **51**:245-251

[41] Bartolucci EG, Swan RH, Hurt WC. Oral manifestations of hereditary hemorrhagic telangiectasia (Osler-Weber-Rendu disease). Journal of Periodontology. 1982;**53**:163-167

[42] da Silva Santos PS, Fernandes KS, Magalhaes MH. Osler-Weber-Rendu syndrome-dental implications. Journal of the Canadian Dental Association. 2009; **75**(7):527-530

[43] Corre P, Perret C, Isidor B, Khonsari RH. A brain abscess following dental extractions in a patient with hereditary hemorrhagic telangiectasia. The British Journal of Oral & Maxillofacial Surgery. 2010;**49**:9-11

[44] Mylona E, Vadala C, Papastamopoulos V, Skoutelis A. Brain abscess caused by enterococcus faecalis following a dental procedure in a patient with hereditary hemorrhagic telangiectasia. Journal of Clinical Microbiology. 2012;**50**(5):1807-1809. DOI: 10.1128/JCM.06658-11

[45] Cartin-Ceba R, Swanson KL, Krowka MJ. Pulmonary arteriovenous malformations. Chest. 2013;**144**(3): 1033-1044. DOI: 10.1378/chest.12-0924

[46] te Veldhuis EC, te Veldhuis AH, van Dijk FS, Kwee ML, van Hagen JM,

Baart JA, et al. Rendu-Osler-Weber disease: Update of medical and dental considerations. Oral Surgery, Oral Medicine, Oral Pathology, Oral Radiology, and Endodontics. 2008; **105**(2):e38-e41. DOI: 10.1016/j.tripleo.2007.08.017

[47] Shovlin C, Bamford K, Sabbà C, Mager HJ, Kjeldsen A, Droege F, et al. Prevention of serious infections in hereditary hemorrhagic telangiectasia: Roles for prophylactic antibiotics, the pulmonary capillaries-but not vaccination. Haematologica. 2019; **104**(2):e85-e86. DOI: 10.3324/haematol.2018.209791

[48] Tessier S, Lipton BA, Ido F, Longo S, Nanda S. Pathogenesis and therapy of arteriovenous malformations: A case report and narrative review. International Journal of Critical Illness and Injury Science. 2021;**11**(3):167-176. DOI: 10.4103/IJCIIS.IJCIIS_127_20. Epub 2021 Sep 25

[49] Dupuis-Girod S, Ginon I, Saurin JC, Marion D, Guillot E, Decullier E, et al. Bevacizumab in patients with hereditary hemorrhagic telangiectasia and severe hepatic vascular malformations and high cardiac output. Journal of the American Medical Association. 2012;**307**:948-955

[50] Derossi SS, Raghavendra S. Anemia. Oral Surgery, Oral Medicine, Oral Pathology, Oral Radiology, and Endodontics. 2003;**95**(2):131-141. DOI: 10.1067/moe.2003.13

[51] Ramirez B, Morais D, Condado MA, et al. A new sclerosant for the treatment of Rendu-Osler-Weber disease. Acta Otorrinolaringológica Española. 2000;**51**: 36-39

[52] Morais D, Ramirez B, Santos J. Local sclerosant treatment with etoxisclerol in ENT pathologies: Rendu-Osler-Weber disease, granulomas, angiomas. Acta Otor-rinolaringológica Española. 2002; **53**:658-661

[53] Morais D, Millás T, Zarrabeitia R, Botella ML, Almaraz A. Local sclerotherapy with polydocanol (Aethoxysklerol®) for the treatment of epistaxis in Rendu-Osler-Weber disease or hereditary hemorrhagic telangiectasia: 15 years of experience. Rhinology. 2012; **50**:80-86

[54] Morais D. Local sclerotherapy with polidocanol (Aethox-ysklerol®) for the treatment of epistaxis in Rendu-Osler-Weber disease or hereditary hemorrhagic tel-angiectasia (HHT). In: Brown ER, editor. Sclerotherapy. Chapter 4. Nova Science Publishers, Inc.; 2014. ISBN: 978-1-63321-619-8

[55] Chitsuthipakorn W, Hoang MP, Kanjanawasee D, Seresi-rikachorn K, Snidvongs K. Treatments of epistaxis in hereditary hemorrhagic telangiectasia: Systematic review and network meta-analysis. Current Allergy and Asthma Reports. 2023;**23**(12):689-701. DOI: 10.1007/s11882-023-01116-8

Chapter 5

Elevated Non-fasting Plasma Total Homocysteine Level is Associated with Alveolar Bone and Tooth Loss: Insights for Osteogenic Innovations

Ziyad S. Haidar

Abstract

Tooth loss can cause functional impairment, in terms of chewing/mastication ability and choice of foods/diet, leading to malnutrition, which might ultimately impact general health and well-being. No studies on homocysteine (Hcy), an inflammatory sulfur-containing amino acid biomarker, levels, and tooth loss (or number of remaining teeth), are present. This study opted to obtain data from the available National Health and Nutrition Examination Survey III (NHANES III) and perform statistical analysis to investigate the association between tooth loss and tHcy (plasma/serum levels), with a focus on the elderly population. Acquired data for 1568 individuals aged 65 years or older were then tabulated, to detail. Age, gender, cholesterol, income, education, exercise, creatinine, systolic blood pressure, body mass index, and dental state were each found to be independently associated with tHcy. In a multiple regression model, only age ($\rho < 0.0001$), education ($\rho < 0.0001$), creatinine ($\rho < 0.0001$), and dental state ($\rho < 0.003$) were significantly associated with tHcy, explaining 22% of the variation detected in log-[tHcy]. Plasma Hcy levels in patients are associated with dental status and can be notably affected with oro-dental health, socioeconomic status, and access to therapeutic interventions. Considering these findings, tHcy level monitoring (to diagnose vitamin B6, B9/folate/folic acid or B12 deficiency) as well as nutritional counseling and vitamin supplementation (rechecked post-8 weeks) should be considered and incorporated into the diagnostic and treatment plan for the edentate/edentulous elders, especially if other cardiovascular or inflammatory risk factors are present. In the context of osteogenesis and oral health, research exploring the relationship between elevated Hcy levels and alveolar bone, and tooth loss can provide valuable insights into the underlying mechanisms of bone metabolism and dental health. Understanding how Hcy levels impact bone density, bone remodeling processes, and periodontal health can potentially lead to the design, innovation, development, and translation of novel therapeutic approaches and preventive strategies for osteoporosis, periodontal disease, as well as tooth loss.

Keywords: edentulism, diet, dentition, geriatric, homocysteine, innovation, socioeconomic status, OHRQoL

1. Introduction

According to the US-CDC (Centers for Disease Control and Prevention, the national public/federal health agency of the United States under the Department of Health and Human Services, headquartered in Atlanta, Georgia), about 1 in 6 (17%) adults aged 65 or older have lost all their teeth (**Figure 1**). Thus far, the two most prevalent oral diseases and causes of tooth loss continue to be caries/decay and periodontal disease. Also, more than 1 in 3 adults aged 65 or older who were from the low-income group, had less than a high school education and were smoking cigarettes (2011–2016) lost all their teeth/dentition. *Severe* tooth was found to be 50% higher in those with fair or poor general health status suffering from asthma, heart disease, diabetes, liver conditions, emphysema, rheumatoid arthritis, and with a history of stroke, when compared to people without these chronic conditions. Indeed, it is today well recognizable that tooth loss and severe tooth loss affect Oral Health-Related Quality of Life (OHRQoL), overall QoL, well-being, successful/comfortable aging, and longevity [1, 2]. All of these factors are thought to be closely associated with the quality of the diet [3]. Further, it is well established that socioeconomic status affects diet and, consequently, QoL and OHRQoL, especially in older people (ρ low intake of certain types of foods, nutrients, and minerals). Logically, a poorer diet (quality) often costs less, and while it might be more energy-dense, and it is often more nutrient-poor [2]. In 2019, Nakamura et al. [4] conducted a cross-sectional analysis of data from 2049 Japanese individuals aged ≥50 years, concluding that having a few/fewer remaining teeth was associated with a low nutrient intake and low serum albumin levels, evident in individuals from the low socioeconomic group (with annual household income of <2 million Japanese yen: estimated at ~14,500 USD; equivalent household expenditure per month). The study emphasized the importance of promoting oral and dental health (as well as dietary strategies) in low-income, middle-aged, and older people to help sustain an adequate nutritional status [4].

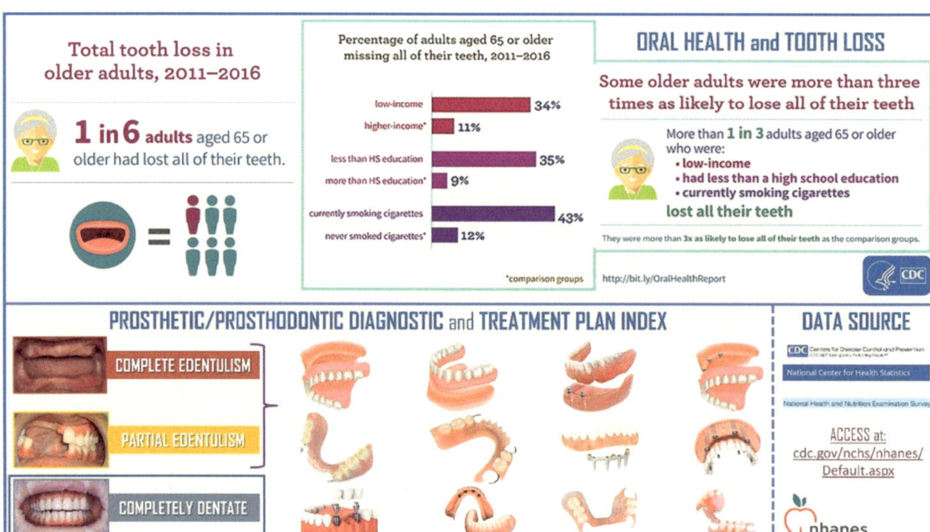

Figure 1.
Geriatric oral health and tooth loss. CDC correlation between tooth loss and socioeconomic factors in the elderly (TOP). Dentition loss classification and traditional treatment options for rehabilitation (BOTTOM-left). Analytical data source: US-CDC/NCHS and laboratory testing included in NHANES III (BOTTOM-right).

Further, severe loss of teeth, particularly complete edentulism, has been associated with the reduced/diminished ability to properly chew/masticate foods (hence leading to a preference for easy-to-consume/-swallow diet that is often richer in fat or dairy products), with poor general health and increased mortality, even when socioeconomic factors are taken into account [5]. Edentulism has indeed been linked to an increase in the prevalence of coronary disease [6, 7], stroke [8], dementia [8, 9], cancer [5], and diabetes [10]. Indeed, almost two decades ago, Joshipura et al. [11, 12] tackled this nutritional state link and found that the average intake of dietary fiber, vegetables, and fruits decreased with the loss of teeth, noting that in parallel, the consumption of calories and saturated fat increased. Similar findings have been reported by other authors and studies [3, 4, 13, 14]. Therefore, it can be stated herein that the impact on QoL and OHRQoL of disease as well as oral and dental rehabilitation (**Figure 1**) and its *termed* (short vs. long) consequences should be taken into consideration when assessing the overall health status and evaluating the clinical outcomes of therapeutics.

Herein, with recent advances in diagnostic technologies and multi-disciplinary strategies, there is accruing evidence that inadequate intake of certain nutrients, even at a level insufficient to cause classical deficiency syndromes, is linked to cardiovascular disease, neural tube defects, and cancer [15]. For example, *plasma homocysteine (tHcy)*, a sulfur-containing amino acid (**Figure 2**), found to be increased/elevated in various inflammatory conditions, can be considered as a functional (inflammatory) biomarker of the nutritional status and a novel and independent risk factor for cardiovascular disease, among others. This is due to the fact that total plasma homocysteine concentration (tHcy) varies with the intake of the group B vitamins, namely folate/folic acid, B12, and B6 [16], making it sensitive to metabolic changes according to or dependent on the intake of fresh fruit, vegetables, and meat [17]. Indeed, higher tHcy levels are associated with increases (risk) in cardiovascular disease, as mentioned earlier, in addition to peripheral artery disease, deep vein thrombosis, renal disease, dementia, and cognitive dysfunction in the elderly [18–20]. For instance, tHcy >14.4 μmol/L is now associated with twice the risk of carotid stenosis when compared with low plasma homocysteine (< 9.1 μmol/L), after correction for other factors [21]. In addition, to simplify to the reader, it has been estimated that an increase in tHcy of 1 μmol/L is associated with a 10% increase in risk of cardiovascular disease [22]. Furthermore, tHcy levels have been correlated with other risk factors and major lifestyle determinants, including gender (male), age, smoking, and

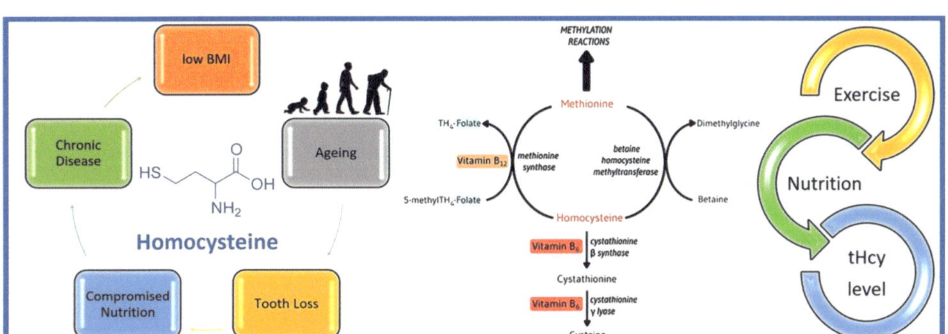

Figure 2.
Homocysteine. Hcy molecular structure, mechanistic pathway, and its role in patient overall health, general well-being, and quality of life (QoL).

consumption of coffee [18]. An evident association with chronic periodontitis (as an inflammatory disease) was recently demonstrated in otherwise systemically healthy individuals. For example, in a case-control hospital-based study involving 85 age- and sex-matched subjects with chronic periodontitis and 91 healthy controls, elevated tHcy was observed in patients/cases [23]. In another recent longitudinal case-control clinical study [24], with a total of 60 patients, tHcy levels (measured by high-performance liquid chromatography analysis) were compared at baseline and 12 weeks post-periodontal (non-surgical) therapy. Interestingly, the mean levels of plasma Hcy were found to be low in the control group, whereas found to be higher in the test group, at baseline [24]. Both tHcy levels and all the detected periodontal parameters were reduced significantly, after intervention, yet were not reduced in cases to levels comparable to controls/periodontally healthy individuals [25]. Nonetheless, for patients at high risk of cardiovascular diseases, for example, periodontal therapy can perhaps be a useful or helpful Hcy-lowering adjunct procedure, worthy of appraisal, *a topic of current research, development, and innovation.*

As depicted in **Figure 2**, and recently reported by Debreceni and Debreceni [25], the group B vitamins do play an essential role in the Hcy metabolism pathway (transformation and excretion: trans-methylation reactions forms Hcy ρ oxidized biomolecule bound to plasma proteins ρ which is then re-methylated back to methionine or is converted into cysteine in trans-sulfuration reactions). For instance, the remethylation reaction requires, among others, vitamin B9 as substrate and vitamin B12 as a co-factor, hence why Hcy can be considered a functional marker for the systemic availability of B9 and B12 [26]. In an edentulous patient, it can be stated that despite advances in rehabilitation, prosthodontics, and dentures, and given ample limitations or hurdles (such as functional/esthetic expertise, availability/accessibility, and cost issues), masticatory/chewing ability is not yet fully or adequately restored. Indeed, a 2018 randomized, cross-over, and double-blinded clinical trial [27] compared, through masticatory tests and a questionnaire, the feeling of retention, stability, and accumulation of particles below the removable denture (complete) among patients with and without adhesives, hypothesizing that the use of adhesives for enhanced retention stability does not increase patient satisfaction with their dentures [27]. Such studies aiming to promote patient experience and satisfaction with removable dentures as a decisive factor in therapeutic or rehabilitative success (with a clear impact on OHRQoL and QoL), continue, especially in low socioeconomic populations, with limited to no access to *superior* implant-supported overdentures [28–30], for example, which have reported significant improvements in masticatory ability and improved nutritional state, yet, to the best of knowledge no studies have investigated correlations with tHcy levels. Further, despite accruing reports focusing on periodontal diseases, none on tooth loss and tHcy were found in the available literature ρ Nakamura et al. [4] investigated serum albumin and hemoglobin levels as the nutritional biomarkers associated with the number of teeth – in quadrants), thus triggering the present analysis.

Herein, data from the National Health and Nutrition Examination Survey III (NHANES III), an accessible and readily available program of health-related studies (one of a series conducted by the CDC and its National Center for Health Statistics or NCHS – oversampling GIS Data/FTP file server; can visit survey methods, sample design, datasets, weighing procedures, analytical guidelines and related documentation at the US Department of Health and Human Services and/or the CDC/NCHS-NHANES (**Figure 1**) combining interviews/questionnaires and physical/clinical/laboratory examinations, designed cross-sectionally to assess the health and nutritional status of adults and children (random sampling selection) in the United States, representative of the non-institutionalized civilian population, was employed to test the hypothesis that tooth loss and edentulism associated with elevated serum homocysteine concentration, in the elderly (> 65 years).

2. Materials and methods

Using the SAS Universal Viewer (SAS Institute Inc., NC, USA), data from male and female individuals of all races who were 65 years or older were included in the analysis, as well as factors known to influence tHcy: age (years), gender (male, female), smoking status, alcohol consumption, serum creatinine levels (mg/dl), total cholesterol (mg/dl), systolic blood pressure (mmHg), socioeconomic status (represented by education and income), coffee consumption, exercise, body mass index (kg/m^2), and dental status. Because our hypothesis was that elevated tHcy might be caused by wearing dentures, the dental status has opted to be defined as binary or dichotomous: teeth in both arches versus no teeth in at least one arch. Definitions of smoking status, alcohol and coffee consumption, education, income, and exercise are obtainable in the 'APPENDIX'.

2.1 Statistical analysis

First, linear regressions of the continuous dependent variable log[tHcy] were carried out on each of the identified potential predictors. Three highly skewed variables – tHcy, creatinine, and income – were logarithmically transformed before inclusion into the statistical examination, analysis, and interpretation. Subsequently, forward selection was employed to construct a multiple linear regression model for log[tHcy] using only those independent variables that were found to be significant in the performed univariate analysis. For sensitivity analysis, the model was also fitted using backward selection, resulting in reassurance that both model-building strategies lead to the same model.

3. Results

The Third National Health and Nutrition Examination Survey (NHANES III) provided data on 2445 males (47%) and 2807 females (53%). **Table 1** summarizes the basic characteristics of the study population. Note that information on the dental state was only available for 1568 subjects. The mean age of those surveyed was 75.7 years, with an average income of $23,200 and less than 10 years of formal education. Mean body mass index (BMI) was 26.6 kg/m^2 (males = 26.1 kg/m^2; females = 26.9 kg/m^2). The table also describes the mean concentrations of cholesterol and creatinine (mg/dl) and mean systolic blood pressure (mmHg). Herein, the variables found to be significantly related to log[tHcy] in the single variable analyses, which used all available observations for each co-variate, were age ($\rho < 0.0001$), gender ($\rho < 0.0001$), cholesterol level ($\rho = 0.0092$), exercise ($\rho < 0.0016$), dental state ($\rho < 0.0001$), log [creatinine] ($\rho < 0.0001$), log of income ($\rho < 0.0001$), education ($\rho < 0.0001$), body mass index ($\rho = 0.006$), and systolic blood pressure ($\rho = 0.0393$), as displayed in **Table 2**. Our forward selection model-building strategy selected only age, education, blood creatinine, and dental state as being significantly associated with log[tHcy]. After exponentiating the model for log[tHcy] to obtain a model for tHcy, the regression

				Percentile				
Variable	**N**	**Mean**	**Standard Error**	**5th**	**25th**	**50th**	**75th**	**95th**
Age (years)	5252	75.74	0.10	65	70	75	81	88
BMI (kg/m^2)	4461	26.6	0.078	19.2	23.0	26.0	29.4	35.7
Education (years)	5171	9.46	0.06	0	7	10	12	16
Poverty income ratio	4493	2.32	0.03	0.58	1.09	1.77	3.00	6.07
Cholesterol (mg/dl)	4178	220.07	0.70	151	189	217	246	296
Creatinine (mg/dl)	4089	1.22	0.01	0.8	1	1.1	1.3	1.8
SBP (mmHg)	4082	142.88	0.32	113	129	141	155	179
Homocysteine (μmol/L)	1723	12.23	0.16	6.3	8.7	10.8	13.9	22.2

Table 1.
NHANES III population characteristics.

Predictor	**ß**	***ρ*-value**
Smoke cigarettes	0.0297	0.34
Age (y)	0.010	<0.0001
Gender (male)	1.75	<0.0001
Log income (poverty ratio)	−0.081	<0.0001
Education (y)	−0.0.0098	<0.0001
Log creatinine	0.66	<0.0001
SBP (mmHg)	0.00096	0.0393
Cholesterol (mg/dl)	−0.00054	0.0092
Exercise	0.071	0.00016
Drank alcohol in the last month	0.00044	0.983
Coffee	−0.00005	0.829
Edentate in at least one arch	0.096	<0.0001

Table 2.
Performed univariate analysis of tHcy predictors.

coefficients were interpretable as a multiplicative effect on tHcy. For every year increase in age from 65, homocysteine levels increase by 0.6%, and a single additional year of education was associated with a 1% reduction in tHcy. As expected, higher levels of creatinine were associated with increased homocysteine levels ($\rho < 0.0001$). Finally, lacking teeth in at least one arch was associated with a 5% increase in tHcy ($\rho = 0.003$). The amount of variation in log[tHcy] explained by the model was $R^2 = 0.22$ or 22% (high-level/↑), as illustrated in **Table 3**. When teeth were present in both arches, tHcy was 11.7 ± 0.2 μmol/l (mean ± standard error). In contrast, the mean level in those lacking teeth, in at least one arch, was 12.7 ± 0.2 μmol/l. Missing teeth may exhibit a dose-response paradigm. While the difference was not statistically significant ($\rho = 0.15$), those missing teeth in only one arch had mean levels of 12.2 ± 0.4 μmol/l, whereas those missing all teeth had mean levels of 12.9 ± 0.3 μmol/l. Herein, the prevalence of hyperhomocysteinemia (> 14 μmol/l) was 20.1% ± 0.55%

A. Predictor		**ß**	***p*-value**
Age (years)		0.0057	<0.0001
Education		−0.0098	<0.0001
Log creatinine		0.63	<0.0001
Edentate in at least one arch *0.22*)		0.052	0.003
B. Dentition Status	***N***	***Percentage (standard error) of hyperhomocysteinemia >14 µmol/L***	***Mean (standard error) µmol/L***
Completely edentate	498	29.3% (0.9)	12.9 (0.3)
Edentate in one arch	217	25.3% (1.3)	12.2 (0.4)
Present teeth	853	20.4% (0.5)	11.7 (0.2)

Table 3.
Performed multivariable analysis of tHcy predictors (A) and the distribution of tHcy levels according to dental status and present teeth (B).

(ρ ± standard error) in those elders with teeth in both arches, 25.3% ± 1.3% in those with teeth in only one arch, and 29.3% ± 0.9% among the completely edentulous.

4. Discussion

Homocysteine is an amino acid found in the blood, and elevated levels of homocysteine have been linked to various health issues, including cardiovascular disease, neurodegenerative disorders, and bone health problems. Herein, the results of this analytical study of the NHANES III database indicated that lacking all teeth in at least one arch is significantly associated with higher plasma homocysteine levels in people over 65 years. To the best of my knowledge, these findings are the first to link edentulousness with a nutritional bio-indicator of systemic health risk. We also found that plasma total homocysteine concentration (tHcy) is negatively associated with the level of education and confirmed that increasing age and plasma creatinine levels are associated with increased tHcy [18]. As described earlier, studies in the general population have revealed that people with tHcy levels between 0 and 6.3 µmol/L (38% of the population) are in the lowest risk category for coronary artery disease. Those with levels of 6.3–10 µmol/L (52%) are at moderate risk, while the 10% with the highest risk have tHcy >10 µmol/L. Based on this scale, only 5% of our study population are low risk while 50% are at high risk, with the edentulous being the most vulnerable. It has been postulated before that the increased risk of arterial disease and its consequences is mediated through the many adverse effects of Hcy on the arterial wall and on the coagulation cascade [31]. If this is true, an intervention that reduces plasma homocysteine could have a strong effect on health, survival, aging, and longevity. Implant overdentures are a good candidate worthy of further investigation in this direction. Indeed, although dentures partially restore appearance and function, it has long been accepted that they are still inadequate replacements for natural dentition [28–30]. Almost two decades ago, Hung *et al.* [32] studied the relationship between tooth loss and changes in the consumption of fruits, vegetables, and nutrients in a large group of male health professionals. They found that those who lost five or more teeth had a significantly greater consumption of poly-unsaturated fat and were also more likely to stop eating apples, pears, and raw carrots (harder to chew). They also, in this JADA report, noted a *temporal* association between tooth loss and detrimental changes in dietary intake. Evidence from other investigations also supported the observations [23, 24]. Edentulous individuals, therefore, exhibit clear changes in food selection patterns that negatively affect nutrition. This change in diet is a plausible explanation for the effect of a significantly higher plasma homocysteine in the edentulous subjects. Both folate and vitamin B6 are found in fruits and vegetables, vitamin B12 is present mainly in meat, and plasma homocysteine rises if these foods are deficient in the diet, as mentioned earlier and evident in the performed analysis. Importantly, the number of people who have lost all of their teeth (by age 65) remains shockingly high in many countries, according to the WHO, which previously reported 26% in the United States, 30% in Canada, and 46% in the United Kingdom. While the incidence has been declining over the last 30 years, the total number of edentulous cases can be expected/projected to continue to rise for many years to come. Indeed, in a report on the future needs for fixed and removable partial dentures in the United States, Douglass and Watson estimated that the need for dentures will increase to 37.9 million in 2020 [33]. It is therefore reasonable to recommend providing this sub-group of patients with better/superior dental prostheses that could aid and facilitate an increased masticatory efficiency, which in turn leads to significant improvements in diet and nutritional state, and thus better OHRQoL and QoL.

5. Conclusion

Research on the association between elevated homocysteine levels and alveolar bone and tooth loss holds significant promise for advancing our understanding of bone metabolism and oral health, and it has the potential to drive innovation in osteogenesis and dental care in the coming years [34–39]. Diet, and its nutritious quality, is closely related to overall health and general well-being, particularly in the elderly. Poor oral and dental health is associated with low intake of certain types of foods, which can often be due to severe loss of teeth and reduced chewing ability. Indeed, while chronic diseases, such as dental caries and periodontal diseases, are also still highly prevalent and further exacerbated by poor food choices, the risk of tooth loss in old age is rendered higher and alarming, requiring rehabilitative intervention. Demand for care is functional, esthetics, and now, associated with risk for systemic and life-threatening diseases. This analytical study revealed that tooth loss and being edentulous are significantly associated with high levels of serum homocysteine, a risk factor for cardiovascular diseases, among others. Elevated homocysteine levels may increase the risk of coronary disease as well as dementia, stroke, and cancer. In light of these new findings, homocysteine monitoring may be invaluable for the geriatric edentulous patient receiving the best possible rehabilitative and prosthodontic/prosthetic care, combined with paying attention to dietary intake, nutritional profiling/counseling, and recommending vitamin (B-complex: vitamin B6, B9/folate/folic acid and B12, if deficient, and *re*check after every 8 weeks) supplements.

6. Closing remarks

The association between elevated non-fasting plasma total homocysteine levels and alveolar bone and tooth loss is indeed an important topic and note-worthy research theme for potential innovations in osteogenesis in the current year of 2024. Indeed, in the context of osteogenesis and oro-dental health, research exploring the relationship between elevated homocysteine levels and alveolar bone and tooth loss can provide valuable insights into the underlying mechanisms of bone metabolism and dental health (including alveolar bone and dentition loss). Understanding how homocysteine levels impact bone density, bone remodeling processes, and periodontal health can potentially lead to the development of new therapeutic approaches and preventive strategies for osteoporosis, periodontal disease, and tooth loss. Furthermore, innovations in osteogenesis may involve novel interventions targeting homocysteine metabolism to promote bone regeneration and prevent bone loss. This could include the development of pharmacological agents, dietary interventions, and personalized treatment approaches aimed at optimizing homocysteine levels and improving bone health outcomes.

Acknowledgements

This work was supported by operating grants provided to the HAiDAR R&D&I LAB/BioMAT'X (Laboratorio de Biomateriales, Farmacéuticos y Bioingeniería de Tejidos Cráneo Máxilo-Facial), member of CiiB (Centro de Investigación e Innovación Biomédica), Faculties of Medicine and Dentistry, Universidad de los Andes, Santiago de Chile, through the ANID-NAM (Agencia Nacional de Investigación y Desarrollo, Chile and National Academy of Medicine, USA) Grant#NAM21I0022, CORFO Crea y Valida I + D + i Grant#21CVC2-183649 and FONDEF CONCURSO IDEA DE I + D, FONDEF/SUBDIRECCIÓN DE INVESTIGACIÓN APLICADA/ANID 2022, Grant código # ID22I10215.

Author contributions

Conceptualization, Validation, Investigation, Resources, Writing – Original Draft Preparation, Writing – Final Manuscript Review and Editing, Funding Acquisition.

Conflict of interest

None.

Appendix A

A.1 Defining the NHANES study variables for present statistical analysis

Smoking status was defined by the binary NHANES variable HAR3, indicating whether the subject smoked cigarettes (at the time), or not. Alcohol consumption was derived from variables HAN6HS, HAN6IS, and HAN6JS. These variables recorded how many drinks of beer, wine, and liquor, respectively, the subject had drunk in the past month. Our derived binary variable simply indicated whether the subject had reported drinking any alcoholic beverages during the past month or not. To examine the socioeconomic status, we looked at education and income separately. Education, defined by the NHANES variable HFA8R, represented the total number of years of education and varied from 0 to 17. Income was analyzed using the variable DMPPIR, which represented the poverty income ratio and was computed by dividing the observed family income category by the poverty threshold. The poverty income ratio was preferred to family income because it allows a valid comparison of the families surveyed during/over the different years. Because this variable was highly skewed, and some individuals had a poverty income ratio of zero, our income variable was defined as log (DMPPIR+1). Coffee consumption, defined by the NHANES variable HAN6FS, reflected the reported number of cups of coffee consumed per month. Physical exercise was, herein, defined by the variables HAT2, HAT4, HAT6, HAT8, HAT10, HAT12, HAT14, and HAT16. Each of these variables recorded whether the subject had engaged in a specific type of activity (for example, jogging, cycling, swimming, and/or gardening) during the past month. Our composite exercise variable simply recorded whether the subject had answered yes to at least one of these activities. The body mass index, defined by the variable BMI, is simply an individual's weight in kilograms divided by his or her squared height in meters. Finally, the tooth loss variable was set to binary. Subjects were considered to be edentulous, if they were missing all of the teeth in one entire arch (or in both arches).

Author details

Ziyad S. Haidar[1,2,3,4,5]

1 BioMAT'X R&D&I (HAiDAR I+D+i LAB), Universidad de los Andes, Chile

2 Facultad de Odontología, Universidad de los Andes, Chile

3 Centro de Investigación e Innovación Biomédica (CiiB), Universidad de los Andes, Chile

4 Facultad de Medicina, Programa de Doctorado en BioMedicina, Universidad de los Andes, Chile

5 Facultad de Odontología, Programa de Doctorado en Ciencias Odontológicas, Universidad de los Andes, Chile

*Address all correspondence to: zhaidar@uandes.cl

References

[1] Marino R, Schofield M, Wright C, Calache H, Minichiello V. Self-reported and clinically determined oral health status predictors for quality of life in dentate older migrant adults. Community Dentistry and Oral Epidemiology. 2008;**36**(1):85-94

[2] Tsakos G, Herrick K, Sheiham A, Watt RG. Edentulism and fruit and vegetable intake in low-income adults. Journal of Dental Research. 2010;**89**(5):462-467

[3] Walls AWG, Steele JG. The relationship between oral health and nutrition in older people. Mechanisms of Ageing and Development. 2004;**125**(12):853-857

[4] Nakamura M, Ojima T, Nagahata T, Kondo I, Ninomiya T, Yoshita K, et al. Having few remaining teeth is associated with a low nutrient intake and low serum albumin levels in middle-aged and older Japanese individuals: Findings from the NIPPON DATA2010. Environmental Health and Preventive Medicine. 2019;**24**(1):1

[5] Abnet CC, Qiao YL, Dawsey SM, Dong ZWPRT, Mark SD. Tooth loss is associated with increased risk of total death and death from upper gastrointestinal cancer, heart disease and stroke in a Chinese population-based cohort. International Journal of Epidemiology. 2005;**34**(2):467-474

[6] Dietrich T, Jimenez M, Krall Kaye EA, Vokonas PS, Garcia RI. Age-dependent associations between chronic periodontitis/edentulism and risk of coronary heart disease. Circulation. 2008;**117**(13):1668-1674

[7] Okoro CA, Balluz LS, Eke PI, Ajani UA, Strine TW, Town M. Tooth loss and heart disease findings from the behavioral risk factor surveillance system. American Journal of Preventive Medicine. 2005;**29**(5):50-56

[8] Joshipura KJ, Hung H, Rimm EB, Willett WC, Ascherio A. Periodontal disease, tooth loss, and incidence of ishchemic stroke. Stroke. 2003;**34**(1):47-52

[9] Lund J, Mojon P, Pho M, Feine J. Alzheimer's disease and edentulism. Age and Ageing. 2003;**32**(2):228-238

[10] Cleary TJ, Hutton JE. An assessment of the association between functional edentulism, obesity, and NIDDM. Diabetes Care. 1995;**18**(7):1007-1009

[11] Joshipura KJ, Willett WC, Douglass CW. The impact of edentulousness on food and nutrient intake. Journal of the American Dental Association (1939). 1996;**127**(4):459-467

[12] Joshipura KJ, Rithchie C, Douglass CW. Strength of evidence linking oral conditions and systemic disease. In: Compendium of Continuing Education in Dentistry. Vol. 30. Jamesburg, NJ; 1995, 2000. pp. 12-23

[13] Krall E, Hayes C, Garcia R. How dentition status and masticatory function affect nutrient intake. Journal of the American Dental Association (1939). 1998;**129**(9):1261-1269

[14] Sheiham A, Steele JG, Marcenes W, Lowe C, Finch S, Bates CJ. The relationship among dental status, nutrient intake, and nutritional status in older people. Journal of Dental Research. 2001;**80**(2):408-413

[15] Mason JB. Biomarkers of nutrient exposure and status in one-carbon

(methyl) metabolism. Journal of Nutrition. 2003;**133**:9415-9475

[16] Maxwell SRJ. Coronary artery disease - free radical damage, antioxidant protection and the role of homocysteine. Basic Research in Cardiology. 2000;**95**(7):I65

[17] Selhub J. Folate, vitamin B12 and vitamin B6 and one carbon metabolism. The Journal of Nutrition, Health & Aging. 2002;**6**(1):39-42

[18] Nygard O, Refsum H, Ueland PM, Vollset SE. Major lifestyle determinants of plasma total homocysteine distribution: The Hordaland homocysteine study. The American Journal of Clinical Nutrition. 1998;**67**(2):263-270

[19] Seshadri S, Beiser A, Selhub J, Jacques PF, Rosenberg IH, D'Agostino RB, et al. Plasma homocysteine as a risk factor for dementia and Alzheimer's disease. The New England Journal of Medicine. 2002;**346**(7):476-483

[20] Seshadri N, Robinson K. Homocysteine, B vitamins, and coronary artery disease. The Medical Clinics of North America. 2000;**84**(1):215-237

[21] Selhub J, Jacques PF, Wilson PW, Rush D, Rosenberg IH. Vitamin status intake as primary determinants of homocysteinemia in an elderly population. JAMA. 1993;**22**(270):2693-2698

[22] Boushey CJ, Beresford SA, Omenn GS, Motulsky AG. A quantitative assessment of plasma homocysteine as a risk factor for vascular disease. Probable benefits of increasing folic acid intake. Journal of the American Medical Association. 1995;**274**(13):1049-1053

[23] Joseph R, Nath SG, Joseraj MG. Elevated plasma homocysteine levels in chronic periodontitis: A hospital-based case-control study. Journal of Periodontology. 2011;**82**(3):439-444

[24] Penmetsa GS, Bhaskar RU, Mopidevi A. Analysis of plasma homocysteine levels in patients with chronic periodontitis before and after nonsurgical periodontal therapy using highperformance liquid chromatography. Contemporary Clinical Dentistry. 2020;**11**:266-273

[25] Debreceni B, Debreceni L. The role of homocysteine-lowering B-vitamins in the primary prevention of cardiovascular disease. Cardiovascular Therapeutics. 2014;**32**:130-138

[26] Herrmann W, Obeid R. Vitamins in the Prevention of Human Diseases; de Gruyter. Berlin, Germany: De Gruyter; 2011. ISBN: 9783110214482, 3110214482

[27] Torres-Sánchez C, Montoya-Salazar V, Torres-Lagares D, Gutierrez-Pérez JL, Jimenez-Castellanos E. Satisfaction in complete denture wearers with and without adhesives: A randomized, crossover, double-blind clinical trial. Journal of Clinical and Experimental Dentistry. 2018;**10**(6):585-590

[28] Haidar ZS. The Association between Ratings of General Satisfaction with Conventional Denture and Preference for Mandibular Implant-Retained Overdentures. Montréal, Québec, Canada: Thesis – MSc Dental Medicine and Oral Health Sciences, McGill University; 2005

[29] Haidar ZS. Complete Removable Dentures (Crds) Vs. Implant Overdentures (Iods): An Analysis of Association between Patient Ratings of General Satisfaction with their CRDs and Treatment Preference for IODs. United Kingdom: LAP Lambert Academic Publishing; 28 Nov 2010

ISBN-10: 9783843376167, ISBN-13: 978-3843376167

[30] Samara SA, Haidar ZS. Re-visiting edentulism: complete removable dentures vs. implant overdentures. Journal of Oral Health and Community Dentistry. 2011;**5**(3):107-109

[31] Spence JD. Homocysteine and stroke prevention: Have the trials settled the issue? International Journal of Stroke. 2006;**1**(4):242-244

[32] Hung. Tooth loss and dietary intake. Journal of the American Dental Association (1939). 2003;**134**(9):1185

[33] Douglass CW, Watson AJ. Future needs for fixed and removable partial dentures in the United States. The Journal of Prosthetic Dentistry. 2002;**87**(1):9

[34] Andreotti F, Burzotta F, Mazza A, Manzoli A, Robinson KAM. Homocysteine and arterial occlusive disease: A concise review. Cardiology. 1999;**44**(4):341-345

[35] Centers for Disease Control and Prevention (CDC). Older Adults and Tooth Loss, Centers for Disease Control and Prevention (CDC). 2020a. Available from: https://www.cdc.gov/oralhealth/infographics/older-adult-tooth-loss-tabs.html

[36] Centers for Disease Control and Prevention (CDC). Severe tooth loss and chronic diseases, Centers for Disease Control and Prevention (CDC). 2020b. Available from: https://www.cdc.gov/oralhealth/infographics/severe-tooth-loss.html

[37] Nowjack-Raymer RE, Sheiham A. Association of edentulism and diet and nutrition in U.S adults. Journal of Dental Research. 2003;**2**(82):123-126

[38] Sahyoun NR, Lin CL, Krall E. Nutritional status of the older adult is associated with dentition status. Journal of the American Dietetic Association. 2003;**103**(1):61-66

[39] Tsakos G, Steele JG, Marcenes W, Walls AW, Sheiham A. Clinical correlates of oral health-related quality of life: Evidence from a national sample of British older people. European Journal of Oral Sciences. 2006;**114**(5):391-395

Chapter 6

Phyto-Nanoparticles in Osteogenesis

Nandita Suresh, Betsy Joseph, Tuomas Waltimo and Sukumaran Anil

Abstract

Phyto-nanoparticles derived from plants are an emerging class of nanomaterials that integrate the versatility of nanotechnology with the therapeutic potential of botanical ingredients. This chapter explores the utility of phyto-nanoparticles in stimulating osteogenesis for applications in bone tissue engineering and regeneration. Plant extracts serve as sustainable nanoparticle building blocks or coatings through green synthesis approaches. Resultant phyto-nanoparticles possess multifunctional capabilities stemming from the bioactive phytochemical components that enable the modulation of osteogenic cells like mesenchymal stem cells and osteoblasts. Diverse phyto-nanoparticles based on green tea, *aloe vera*, curcumin, and other plant derivatives have demonstrated the ability to enhance osteoblast differentiation, proliferation, and mineralized matrix deposition. Proposed mechanisms encompass direct cell interactions, sustained intracellular delivery of osteogenic drugs, and complementary anti-inflammatory effects. Capitalizing on these osteogenic properties, researchers have designed innovative tissue engineering scaffolds, functionalized bone implants, and developed therapeutic carriers for diseases like osteoporosis using phyto-nanotechnology. Further innovations in fabrication strategies and integration with emerging technologies will realize smarter, personalized plant-based nanosystems to advance bone regeneration capabilities dramatically.

Keywords: phyto-nanoparticles, osteogenesis, bone tissue engineering, green synthesis, mesenchymal stem cells

1. Introduction

Nanotechnology is a boundless frontier where science and engineering merge to revolutionize the manipulation and fabrication of materials and devices on a minuscule scale, a billionth of a meter [1]. One prominent arena in which it has permeated is medicine, giving rise to nanomedicine, which has endless possibilities in diagnostics, drug delivery, bone, and tissue regeneration. Nanomedicine utilizes the advancement, composition, assessment, and utilization of nano-sized materials and devices to detect and treat various illnesses—from cancer to heart disease to neurological disorders [2]. Nanoparticles can interact specifically with cells and tissues at the molecular level to provide accurate, potent, and long-lasting diagnoses and therapies.

Bone has an innate capacity to regenerate following trauma or disease. However, this self-healing ability is limited to minor defects and often fails for critical segmental losses arising from fracture nonunion, tumor resections, and skeletal abnormalities. Osteogenesis mediated by osteogenic cells drives bone healing and regeneration [3]. Mesenchymal stem cells (MSCs) stimulated by osteoinductive signals can differentiate into osteoblasts, representing the critical bone-forming cell population. Osteoblasts produce extracellular matrix proteins like collagen I and osteocalcin, constituting the organic matrix. Calcium deposition then forms mineralization and complex tissue formation [4]. Incorporating osteogenic cells with supportive biomaterial scaffolds enables engineered bone graft substitutes that integrate seamlessly with host vasculature and tissues after implantation. Beyond functioning as mechanical supports, biomaterial matrices provide biophysical and biochemical cues that direct survival, proliferation, and differentiation [5]. However, clinical translation needs to be improved by non-optimal scaffold properties, leading to poor cell integration and vascularization. There is tremendous scope for novel nanotechnology solutions to address these limitations in scaffold design [6]. Studies have shown that various nanoparticles, including hydroxyapatite, metallic, and rare earth nanoparticles, can support bone growth and enhance the osteogenic differentiation of mesenchymal stem cells [7]. Additionally, researchers have been investigating nanocomposite scaffolds, nanofibers, and nanoparticle-modified polymeric materials to improve tissue engineering scaffolds' physical and chemical properties, ultimately improving osteogenesis [8].

Phyto-nanoparticles are an emerging class of nanoparticles synthesized from bioactive phytochemical (plant-derived) compounds. Ranging from 1 to 100 nm in size, these plant-inspired nanomaterials integrate the physicochemical versatility of nanoscale materials with the vast compositional diversity and therapeutic utility of botanical ingredients [9]. Phyto-nanoparticles encompass nanomaterials derived from edible and medicinal plants, including herbs, fruit and vegetable crop produce, and general botanicals. Phytochemicals are the primary building blocks or functionalizing coatings for engineering nanoparticle architectures through bottom-up self-assembly and surface modification strategies [10].

2. Materials and methods: Literature review and reference selection

This chapter on "Phyto-Nanoparticles in Osteogenesis" was meticulously assembled through a comprehensive literature review using various scientific databases, including PubMed, Scopus, and Web of Science. Search terms used involved combinations of keywords such as "phyto-nanoparticles," "osteogenesis," "bone regeneration," "green synthesis," and "plant extracts." The initial search produced a substantial number of research articles, which were subsequently screened for relevance, with a preference for studies published within the last 5 to 10 years to ensure the inclusion of the latest research developments. Additionally, significant consideration was given to the impact factor of the journals to prioritize high-quality, peer-reviewed sources such as original research articles, review papers, and book chapters. The selected references were thoroughly examined to extract critical data concerning the types of phyto-nanoparticles, their synthesis methods, mechanisms of action, and applications in bone tissue engineering and regeneration. The chapter is structured to offer a detailed overview of the subject, beginning with an introduction to phyto-nanoparticles and their benefits. This is followed by an in-depth discussion on various phyto-nanoparticles, detailing their synthesis, properties, and roles in bone regeneration. References are meticulously integrated throughout the chapter to bolster the information presented and guide readers to further detailed resources for expanded research.

3. Phyto-nanoparticles

Phyto-nanoparticles, synthesized from plant extracts, have garnered considerable attention for their distinctive properties and wide range of potential uses in fields such as medicine, agriculture, and food production. These nanoparticles are environmentally friendly and cost-effective, and their scalability adds to their appeal as a method for synthesizing metal and metal oxide nanoparticles [11]. A multitude of methods are utilized for their synthesis. One such method is phytosynthesis, where plant extracts are employed as both environmentally friendly reducing and capping agents to create metal oxide nanoparticles [12]. Another approach is green synthesis, which harnesses plant extracts, fungi, and algae biomolecules to produce nanoparticles. Biogenic synthesis is highly regarded for its environmentally friendly nature, cost-effectiveness, and potential for easy scalability [9, 13]. Another approach to producing nanoparticles is through seed-mediated synthesis, which utilizes plant seeds. For instance, nanoparticles have successfully been synthesized using fenugreek seed extract [14]. Additionally, the Microwave-assisted method leverages microwave technology to expedite the synthesis of nanoparticles using plant extracts [15]. Ultrasonication involves accelerating nanoparticle synthesis using plant extracts [16]. The FDA has classified plant-based nanoparticles as generally recognized as safe (GRAS) and biodegradable, making them superior to other nanoparticle options for several reasons. They have lower toxicity levels and possess beneficial qualities such as greater energy efficiency and antioxidant, antifungal, antibacterial, and anticancer properties. The use of plant extracts to produce these nanoparticles is believed to contribute to these advantageous properties [17].

3.1 Phyto-nanoparticles in biomedical applications

Phyto-nanoparticles are derived from various plant sources and offer potential drug delivery, imaging, and therapy applications. One of the primary advantages of Phyto-nanoparticles is their biocompatibility and low toxicity compared to synthetic nanoparticles [18]. Plant-based nanoparticles are naturally derived and have a lower risk of causing adverse reactions in the human body. They are also biodegradable, which means they can be easily eliminated from the body after serving their purpose. This makes them an attractive alternative to conventional nanoparticles, which may have potential long-term toxicity concerns. Phyto-nanoparticles can be synthesized from various plant sources, including leaves, fruits, seeds, and roots. The synthesis process typically involves the extraction of plant compounds, followed by reducing and stabilizing metal ions to form nanoparticles [19]. Green synthesis methods, such as using plant extracts as reducing and capping agents, have gained popularity due to their simplicity, cost-effectiveness, and environmental friendliness.

One of the most promising applications of Phyto-nanoparticles in biomedicine is drug delivery (**Figure 1**). Plant-based nanoparticles can be engineered to encapsulate and deliver drugs to specific target sites in the body, improving therapeutic efficacy and reducing side effects [20]. Curcumin, a natural compound found in turmeric, has

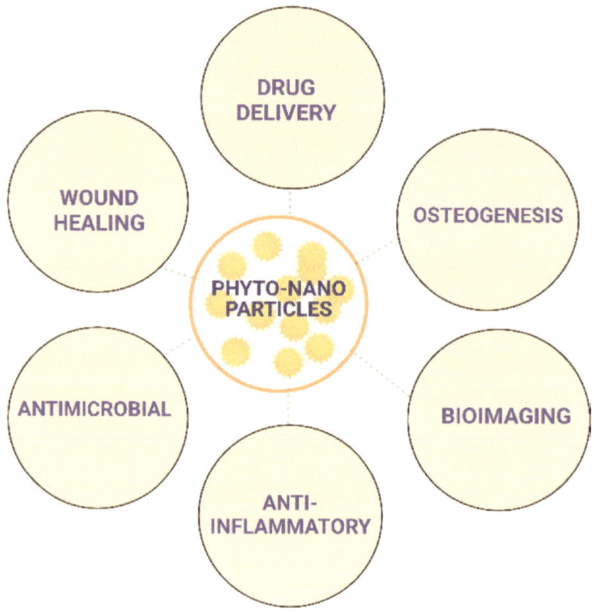

Figure 1.
Biomedical applications of phyto-nanoparticles.

been encapsulated in phyto-nanoparticles derived from various plant sources, such as ginger and *aloe vera*. These nanoformulations have shown enhanced bioavailability, stability, and targeted delivery of curcumin to cancer cells, demonstrating their potential in cancer therapy [21].

In addition to drug delivery, phyto-nanoparticles have also been explored for their potential in imaging and diagnosis. Nanoparticles derived from plants such as tea, grapes, and pomegranate have been found to exhibit fluorescent properties, making them suitable for bioimaging applications [22]. These nanoparticles can be functionalized by targeting ligands to label and image diseased cells or tissues, aiding in the early detection and diagnosis of diseases such as cancer. Moreover, phyto-nanoparticles have shown promise in wound healing and tissue regeneration. Plant-based nanoparticles, such as those derived from *aloe vera* and ginger, have been found to possess antimicrobial and anti-inflammatory properties [23]. When incorporated into wound dressings or scaffolds, these nanoparticles can promote faster wound healing, reduce the risk of infection, and stimulate tissue regeneration.

Phyto-nanoparticlesare promising in biomedical applications due to their biocompatibility, low toxicity, and versatile properties. With their potential in drug delivery, imaging, and therapy, plant-based nanoparticles offer a sustainable and effective alternative to conventional nanoparticles. As research in this field advances, Phyto-nanoparticles are expected to play an increasingly important role in developing novel biomedical technologies for diagnosing and treating various diseases.

3.2 Advantages of plant-based nanoparticles

The growing utilization of plant sources for nanoparticle fabrication is motivated by their unique advantages:

3.2.1 Sustainability

Using plant sources for nanoparticle fabrication offers a more sustainable and environmentally friendly approach than conventional processes. By avoiding toxic chemicals, phyto-nanoparticle synthesis minimizes the negative environmental impact associated with traditional nanoparticle production. This green approach reduces the generation of hazardous waste and the consumption of non-renewable resources. Using plant-based materials also contributes to the renewable nature of phyto-nanoparticle synthesis, as plants can be cultivated and harvested sustainably, ensuring a continuous supply of raw materials without depleting natural resources. Furthermore, the biodegradability of plant-derived nanoparticles reduces the risk of long-term accumulation in the environment, mitigating potential ecological concerns. Overall, the sustainability advantages of plant-based nanoparticle fabrication align with the growing global emphasis on green chemistry and sustainable manufacturing practices, making it an attractive approach for developing eco-friendly nanomaterials [24].

3.2.2 Biocompatibility

The inherent biocompatibility of plant-based nanoparticles is a significant advantage that facilitates their application in biomedical fields. Plants have evolved to produce a wide range of biomolecules that are intrinsically compatible with human physiology, as many of these compounds are naturally present in our diets. When nanoparticles are synthesized using plant extracts, the biocompatibility of the plant components is transferred to the resulting nanomaterials. Plant-derived biomolecules on the surface of the nanoparticles can also enhance their interaction with cells and tissues, promoting better integration and reducing the likelihood of immune rejection. Moreover, the biodegradability of plant-based nanoparticles ensures that they can be safely metabolized and eliminated from the body after serving their therapeutic purpose, minimizing the potential for long-term accumulation and associated health risks [25]. The biocompatibility of phyto-nanoparticles is particularly advantageous for applications such as drug delivery, tissue engineering, and wound healing, where the nanomaterials are intended to interact closely with living systems. By leveraging the inherent biocompatibility of plant-derived materials, researchers can develop safer and more effective nanomedicines and biomedical devices.

3.2.3 Multifunctionality

One of the critical advantages of plant-based nanoparticles is their multifunctionality, which arises from the diverse range of phytochemicals present in plant extracts. Plants produce many bioactive compounds, including polyphenols, flavonoids, alkaloids, and terpenoids, each with unique therapeutic properties. When these phytochemicals are incorporated into nanoparticles, they impart additional functionalities beyond the basic properties of the nanomaterial itself. Furthermore, encapsulating phytochemicals into nanoparticles can improve their stability, protecting them from degradation and enabling controlled release over an extended period. This enhanced stability and sustained release profile can significantly improve encapsulated compounds' bioavailability and therapeutic efficacy [26]. The multifunctional nature of phyto-nanoparticles opens up exciting opportunities for developing targeted therapies and multifaceted approaches to address complex medical challenges.

3.2.4 Scalability

The scalability of plant-based nanoparticle production is another significant advantage that makes it an attractive approach for large-scale manufacturing. Plants can be easily cultivated and harvested in large quantities through well-established agricultural practices, providing an abundant and renewable source of raw materials for nanoparticle synthesis. This scalability is crucial for meeting the increasing demand for nanomaterials in various industrial and biomedical applications. Compared to other methods of nanoparticle production, such as chemical synthesis or microbial fermentation, plant-based approaches offer the potential for higher yields and more cost-effective production. Advances in bioengineering and molecular pharming techniques can further enhance the scalability of phyto-nanoparticle production. For example, genetic engineering can develop transgenic plants that overexpress specific phytochemicals of interest, leading to higher yields of the desired compounds. Similarly, optimization of plant growth conditions and extraction processes can improve the efficiency and productivity of nanoparticle synthesis. The ability to scale up plant-based nanoparticle production is particularly relevant for applications that require large quantities of nanomaterials, such as environmental remediation, agricultural interventions, and industrial catalysis. The scalability of phyto-nanoparticle production and the sustainability and cost-effectiveness of plant-based approaches make it a promising avenue for commercially developing nanomaterials.

These integral advantages underpin the promise of plant-based nanoparticle systems to provide sustainable, therapeutic alternatives to conventional nanomaterials. Phyto-nanoparticles constitute a versatile platform to harness the functional benefits of nanotechnology for human healthcare applications [27].

3.3 Disadvantages and limitations of phyto-nanoparticles

Phyto-nanoparticles, synthesized primarily through green synthesis methods using plant extracts, represent a novel class of nanomaterials that combine nanoparticles' physicochemical properties with plants' biological attributes. Despite their burgeoning application in the biomedical field, several significant limitations and disadvantages persist, impacting their practical utility and efficacy. One primary concern with phyto-nanoparticles is their complex and often inconsistent synthesis process. While green synthesis is touted for its environmental friendliness, the lack of control over the nanoparticles' size, shape, and dispersity can result in varied functional properties. This heterogeneity can adversely affect the reproducibility of experimental results and the scalability of production processes [28]. The biological pathways involved in synthesizing phyto-nanoparticles depend heavily on the type of plant extract used, which can introduce variability due to differences in the plants' concentration and composition of bioactive compounds. These variations make standardizing practices and achieving consistent nanoparticle traits challenging and critical for specific applications, particularly in drug delivery and therapeutic roles.

Moreover, the long-term stability and storage of phyto-nanoparticles pose another significant challenge. Nanoparticles derived from plant sources may be prone to aggregation or degradation over time, diminishing their effectiveness and shelf life. Environmental factors such as temperature, light, and humidity can further exacerbate these stability issues, necessitating sophisticated and often expensive storage solutions to maintain their functional integrity over time [29]. The safety and biocompatibility of phyto-nanoparticles, although generally favorable compared to synthetic nanoparticles, remain areas of concern. The interaction of phyto-nanoparticles with cells and biological systems can sometimes induce cytotoxic effects, particularly at higher concentrations or prolonged exposure. The presence of residual plant materials or contaminants from the synthesis process can also provoke immune responses or inflammatory reactions, which are detrimental in biomedical applications. Additionally, the metabolic pathways involved in degrading and eliminating these nanoparticles from the body are poorly understood, raising concerns about potential bioaccumulation and toxicity [30].

Regulatory challenges also constitute a significant disadvantage. The nanoparticle approval process is stringent and complex, particularly in food and medicine. Phyto-nanoparticles, due to their novel nature, face numerous hurdles in gaining regulatory approval across different jurisdictions. The lack of standardized characterization methods for these nanoparticles further complicates their assessment, requiring extensive and comprehensive studies to establish their safety profiles and therapeutic efficacy. From an application perspective, while phyto-nanoparticles are explored for their potential in various therapeutic and diagnostic roles, their real-world applications are limited by the current understanding of their interactions at the molecular, cellular, and systemic levels. Incomplete knowledge about the mechanisms these nanoparticles exert their effects can limit their design and functional optimization for specific applications. For instance, in drug delivery, the unpredictable release profiles and interaction with biological membranes can result in suboptimal therapeutic outcomes. While phyto-nanoparticles offer several promising advantages, their practical application is hindered by significant limitations related to synthesis variability, stability, safety, regulatory challenges, and incomplete understanding of their biological interactions [31]. Addressing these challenges requires coordinated research efforts to standardize synthesis methods, establish robust safety evaluations, and enhance the functional properties of these nanomaterials for reliable and practical use across various domains.

4. Types of phyto-nanoparticles in osteogenesis

A vast library of plants encompassing food crops, herbs, and their molecular constituents have been transformed into nanocarriers and nanostructures for stimulating stem cell osteogenesis (**Figure 2**). The rich phytochemical reservoirs serve as building elements for nanoparticle synthesis and confer biofunctional outputs [32]. When appropriately engineered into nanosystems, unique properties emerge from the crosstalk between physicochemical and biological cues that effectively direct bone healing.

4.1 Green tea extract nanoparticles

Green tea, derived from the leaves of the *Camellia sinensis* plant, has been identified for its numerous benefits. Its high concentration of polyphenolic compounds, specifically catechins, contributes to its antioxidant, anti-inflammatory, and osteogenic activity [33]. Research has proven that tea extract provides considerable safety in preventing neurodegenerative diseases, including Parkinson's and Alzheimer's [34]. Additionally, green tea has displayed anti-diabetic properties in animal models [35]. Its antibacterial, anti-HIV, anti-aging, and anti-inflammatory activities have also been documented.

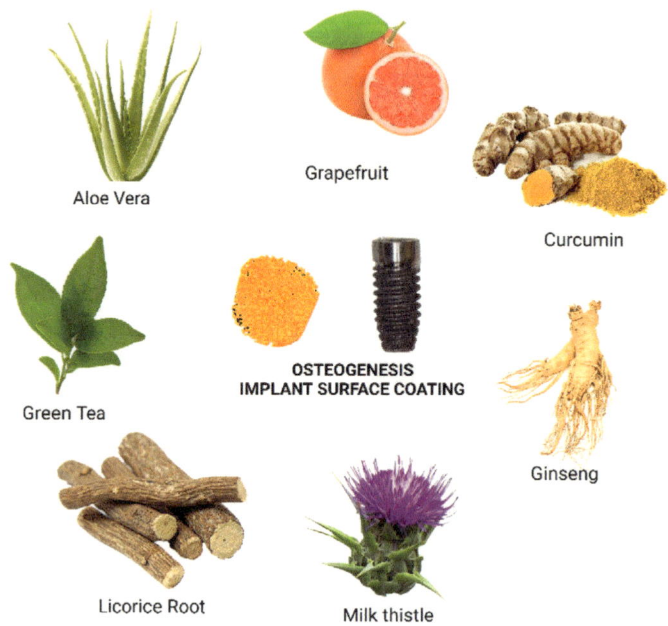

Figure 2.
Diverse plant sources for deriving phyto-nanoparticles with osteogenic potential. Phyto-nanoparticles synthesized from various botanical ingredients, including green tea, aloe vera, curcumin, licorice, flavonoids, silymarin, and ginseng, have shown the ability to stimulate osteoblast activity and bone formation. The rich phytochemical composition of these plant sources confers biofunctional properties to the engineered nanoparticles for directing stem cell differentiation and modulating bone cell fates toward enhanced osteogenesis.

Green tea extract nanoparticles (GTE-NPs) have been shown to have anti-inflammatory effects in animal models. Inflammation is a critical protective mechanism in the healing process. Still, it can also cause pain and swelling associated with pro-inflammatory cytokines such as interleukin (IL) IL-1, IL-6, and tissue necrosis factor-alpha (TNF-α) [36]. GTE-NPs can improve mice's physiological motor and cognitive function during inflammation, indicating their potential therapeutic applications. They also have antioxidant properties, which can help protect cells from oxidative stress and promote tissue regeneration [33].

GTE-NPs offer potential benefits in bone regeneration due to their unique properties, including antioxidant, anti-inflammatory, and osteogenic effects. Green tea has been reported to promote tissue remodeling and bone healing, making it a promising candidate for enhancing bone regeneration [36]. The catechin (−)-epigallocatechin-3-gallate (EGCG) in green tea facilitates fracture healing and increases bone mineral density, indicating its potential to improve bone health [37]. EGCG enhances the osteogenic differentiation of human bone marrow mesenchymal stem cells through the Wnt signaling pathway, which controls bone development. Additionally, green tea catechins enhance osteogenesis in bone marrow mesenchymal stem cells [38]. Animal experiments have indicated that green tea extract EGCG can significantly stimulate bone regeneration in rat skull defects [39]. Furthermore, GTE-NPs combined with hydroxyapatite create composite materials that exhibit favorable bone regeneration abilities [40]. Potential mechanisms of GTE-NPs in promoting osteogenesis include activation of the Wnt pathway, osteogenic differentiation enhancement, and bone regeneration stimulation [41]. Further research is needed to understand the mechanisms of GTE-NPs in osteogenesis fully, but current findings suggest their potential therapeutic applications for bone regeneration and tissue engineering.

4.2 *Aloe vera*-based nanoparticles

Aloe vera, a succulent plant species, has been widely recognized for its diverse medicinal applications. The use of *aloe vera* dates back thousands of years, and its therapeutic properties have been extensively studied. *Aloe vera* is commonly used topically to treat various skin conditions, including burns, cuts, insect bites, and eczemas, owing to its anti-inflammatory, antimicrobial, and wound-healing properties [42]. Additionally, *aloe vera* has been investigated as a dietary supplement, with studies suggesting benefits such as reduced dental plaque, accelerated wound healing, and potential glycemic control [43]. Furthermore, oral *aloe vera* gel has been associated with lowering blood glucose and cholesterol levels, making it attractive for managing diabetes and hyperlipidemia [44]. The plant's unique properties have also led to research on its potential as a cytotoxic, antitumoral, anticancer, and anti-diabetic agent.

Aloe vera promotes wound healing at the cellular and subcellular levels. It accelerates wound healing by stimulating the proliferation and migration of fibroblasts and keratinocytes, which are essential for repairing injured tissues [45]. *Aloe vera* nanoparticles (AVNPs) are a recent development in nanotechnology and have gained attention due to their potential biomedical applications. AVNPs have exhibited the potential to promote osteogenesis owing to their unique antioxidant, anti-inflammatory, and osteogenic effects [46]. Gold nanoparticles (AuNPs) synthesized using *aloe vera* possess osteoinductive properties crucial for bone formation. Using *aloe vera* in AuNP synthesis provides an eco-friendly and cost-effective approach.

Electrophoretic Deposition of *aloe vera*-chitosan-hydroxyapatite nanocomposite coatings onto titanium implants was studied [47]. Chitosan was the binding agent, while hydroxyapatite facilitated osseointegration with surrounding bone. *Aloe vera* particles conferred antibacterial effects against common pathogens like *S. aureus*, responsible for many implant-associated infections. Excellent biocompatibility was verified by the growth and ALP activity of cultured osteosarcoma cells, making this nanocomposite coating ideal for enhancing the functionality of titanium bone implants. Beyond direct osteogenic stimulation, *aloe vera* nanoparticles can also play auxiliary roles, such as anti-scarring during bone healing [48]. *Aloe vera* nanoparticles into a putty containing bioactive glass ceramics and applied as a protective barrier membrane over bone defects. The released *aloe vera* phytochemicals were found to inhibit myofibroblast differentiation and activity of human dermal fibroblasts via TGF-β1 modulation, thus reducing scar tissue formation while permitting unimpeded bone formation across the defect.

4.3 Curcumin nanoparticles

Curcumin is a chemical compound found in the *Curcuma longa* plant, also known as turmeric. It is a popular condiment with antioxidant, anti-inflammatory, antimicrobial, and anticancer properties, and it has been widely used in indigenous and traditional medicine [27]. Research suggests that curcumin may help manage oxidative stress, inflammation, metabolic syndrome, arthritis, anxiety, and degenerative eye diseases [49].

In vitro and in vivo studies have demonstrated anti-inflammatory, anti-diabetic, anti-proliferative, and pro-apoptotic effects against various tumors [50]. Curcumin has also exhibited potential against Alzheimer's, multiple sclerosis, rheumatoid arthritis, atherosclerosis, cataracts, liver damage, lung toxicity, fibrosis, bleeding, clotting, platelet aggregation, and wound healing. However, more bioavailability is needed to ensure its maximal therapeutic potential. Strategies to improve bioavailability include adjuvants like piperine, lipid formulations, structural analogs, and nanoparticulate delivery systems using natural and synthetic polymer-based carriers [51, 52]. These approaches enhance curcumin's solubility, stability, and absorption to maximize its efficacy.

Nanoparticles of curcumin, also known as nano curcumin, have been extensively researched for improving bioavailability and therapeutic effects. Wet-milling, nanoprecipitation, and other techniques produce nano curcumin with reduced particle size and increased solubility. One study described wet-milled nano curcumin with a narrow size distribution [53], while another emphasized green manufacturing approaches to improve curcumin bioaccessibility [54]. Nanocurcumin formulations have improved efficacy and bioavailability in vivo, making them promising for cancer therapy [55]. Curcumin nanoparticles also have potential applications in dental implantology owing to their antibacterial properties against pathogens like *Porphyromonas gingivalis*, which commonly cause implant failure [56]. In conclusion, curcumin nanoparticles represent a promising means to enhance the therapeutic potential of curcumin through improved bioavailability and antimicrobial activity. Further research and clinical studies are essential to fully realize their potential while ensuring safety and efficacy for medical and dental uses.

Scaffold fabrication using the curcumin/graphene oxide/hydroxyapatite nanoparticles resulted in sustained curcumin release over a month. Analysis with osteoblast-like MG-63 cells revealed significant upregulation of osteogenic markers like osteopontin and bone sialoprotein compared to pure hydroxyapatite controls, confirming the critical role of released curcumin in driving differentiation [57].

4.4 Other plant-derived nanoparticles

In addition to the well-studied green tea extract, *aloe vera*-based, and curcumin nanoparticles, researchers have explored numerous lesser-known but promising plant-derived nanoparticles for stimulating bone regeneration. The diverse range of plant-derived nanoparticles presents a promising frontier in osteogenesis. Their unique properties, including bioactivity, biocompatibility, and biodegradability, make them suitable candidates for enhancing bone regeneration and treating bone-related diseases.

4.4.1 Grapefruit extract nanoparticles

Grapefruit extract contains naringin, a flavonoid with antioxidative and anti-inflammatory activities. Naringin nanoparticles promoted osteogenic differentiation of mesenchymal stem cells (MSCs) by upregulating bone morphogenetic protein-2 (BMP-2) and suppressing nuclear factor-kB (NF-kB) [58]. This photo-nanoparticle also increased alkaline phosphatase (ALP) activity, stimulated collagen production, and deposited calcium. Its ability to dually promote osteogenesis and inhibit osteoclastogenesis makes it a promising agent for restoring bone defects [59].

4.4.2 Licorice root nanoparticles

Licorice is a popular herbal medicine containing glabridin, which has estrogenic effects and helps manage postmenopausal osteoporosis. Glabridin nanoparticles enhanced viability and osteogenic differentiation in MSCs by stimulating estrogen receptor signaling [60]. It also inhibited hydrogen peroxide-induced cytotoxicity and reactive oxygen species production. As a phytoestrogen, glabridin is safer than traditional hormone replacement therapy for osteoporosis [61].

4.4.3 Flavonoid nanoparticles

Flavonoids, a diverse group of phytonutrients found in almost all fruits and vegetables, exhibit strong antioxidant properties. The encapsulation of flavonoids into nanoparticles has been explored to enhance their bioavailability and efficacy in osteogenesis [62]. For instance, when formulated into nanoparticles, quercetin, a well-known flavonoid, has significantly improved osteoblast proliferation and differentiation [63]. The enhanced solubility and stability of quercetin nanoparticles facilitate their uptake by bone cells, thereby stimulating the expression of osteogenic markers such as alkaline phosphatase (ALP), osteocalcin, and bone morphogenetic proteins (BMPs).

4.4.4 Silymarin nanoparticles

Silymarin, derived from the milk thistle plant (*Silybum marianum*), is another phytochemical with potent antioxidant and anti-inflammatory properties. Silymarin nanoparticles have been investigated for their potential in osteogenesis due to their ability to modulate bone metabolism [64]. Studies have demonstrated that silymarin nanoparticles can enhance osteoblasts' proliferation and mineralization while inhibiting osteoclasts' formation and activity. By balancing the activities of these cells, silymarin nanoparticles contribute to the maintenance and regeneration of bone tissue, making them a promising candidate for bone tissue engineering and the treatment of osteoporosis [65].

4.4.5 Ginseng nanoparticles

Ginseng, a traditional herbal medicine, contains bioactive compounds called ginsenosides, which have been implicated in various therapeutic effects, including osteogenesis. Ginsenoside-loaded nanoparticles have been designed to overcome the poor bioavailability of ginsenosides, enhancing their therapeutic potential in bone health [66]. These nanoparticles stimulate osteoblast differentiation and bone formation by activating the Wnt/β-catenin signaling pathway. Furthermore, ginseng nanoparticles have been shown to exert immunomodulatory effects, which can significantly benefit conditions characterized by inflammation-induced bone loss, such as osteoporosis and rheumatoid arthritis.

5. Mechanisms of action

Elucidating the mechanistic pathways involved in augmented osteogenic stimulation by phyto-nanoparticles remains an intense research pursuit. Uncovering these mechanisms at the biomolecular and cellular levels provides design feedback better to tailor nanoparticle properties for their intended modulatory roles. Central operating mechanisms encompass direct interactions of the nanoparticles with osteogenic cells to alter differentiation or activity, sustained intracellular delivery of cargo osteogenic drugs, and auxiliary anti-inflammatory and antimicrobial functionality.

The **Table 1** summarizes the key processes through which each phyto-nanoparticle influences bone formation and remodeling. These mechanisms include the stimulation of osteoblast differentiation and mineralization, inhibiting osteoclast formation and activity, and modulation of signaling pathways involved in bone metabolism, such as Wnt/β-catenin, RANKL/OPG, BMP, and MAPK. The phyto-nanoparticles listed in the table are flavonoids, curcumin, resveratrol, quercetin, epigallocatechin gallate (EGCG), daidzein, and genistein. It is important to note that each phytonanoparticle may exert its effects through multiple cellular and molecular mechanisms, collectively contributing to the overall process of osteogenesis.

5.1 Interaction with osteoblasts and osteoclasts

Plant nanoparticles have potential applications in bone remodeling, particularly on osteoblasts and osteoclasts. The studies suggest that the bioactive effects of

Phyto-nanoparticle	Mechanism of Action in Osteogenesis
Flavonoids	• Stimulate osteoblast differentiation and mineralization • Inhibit osteoclast formation and activity • Enhance bone formation markers (e.g., alkaline phosphatase, collagen)
Curcumin	• Promotes osteoblast differentiation and mineralization • Suppresses osteoclastogenesis and bone resorption • Modulates Wnt/β-catenin signaling pathway
Resveratrol	• Enhances osteoblast differentiation and bone formation • Inhibits osteoclast differentiation and activity • Activates SIRT1 and AMPK signaling pathways
Quercetin	• Stimulates osteoblast proliferation and differentiation • Inhibits osteoclast formation and bone resorption • Modulates RANKL/OPG ratio
Epigallocatechin gallate (EGCG)	• Promotes osteoblast differentiation and mineralization • Suppresses osteoclast differentiation and activity • Regulates BMP and MAPK signaling pathways
Daidzein	• Enhances osteoblast proliferation and differentiation • Inhibits osteoclastogenesis and bone resorption • Activates estrogen receptor signaling
Genistein	• Stimulates osteoblast differentiation and bone formation • Suppresses osteoclast formation and activity • Modulates TGF-β/BMP and Wnt/β-catenin signaling pathways

Table 1.
Mechanisms of action of various Phyto-nanoparticles in osteogenesis.

nanoparticles on bone cells are size, surface property, and composition-dependent. For instance, silica nanoparticles have been demonstrated to improve bone mass and promote the differentiation of bone cells. Similarly, metallic nanoparticles are viable alternatives for bone repair and regeneration due to their bioactivity, biomimetic composition, and good incorporation within the natural bone structure [67]. Orchestrating the coordinated actions of bone-forming osteoblasts and resorbing osteoclasts is critical to developing mature mineralized tissues (**Figure 3**). Phyto-nanoparticles influence osteogenic outcomes through direct contact with these cells to modulate lineage commitment, differentiation, proliferation, adhesion, and matrix deposition. Particle internalization enables intracellular cargo delivery, while surface coatings present instructive cues to direct cell fate [68]. Nanotopography-mediated contact guidance is emerging as a powerful approach to control stem cell differentiation trajectories. Using green tea polyphenol nanoparticles, Luo et al. [69] described enhanced adhesion, spread, and proliferation in rat mesenchymal stem cells, which correlated with osteogenic marker expression. They postulated that the nanoparticle surfaces provided nanoscale cues resembling fibrillar bone extracellular matrix to promote osteoblastic phenotypes. Inorganic nanoparticles like hydroxyapatite similarly stimulated the fibroblastic differentiation of pre-osteoblastic MC3T3-E1 cells [70].

Iron oxide nanoparticles have been shown to promote osteoblast differentiation and inhibit osteoclast activity, suggesting a potential role in bone remodeling and regeneration [71]. Iron oxide nanoparticles can be synthesized using plant extracts, which offer a cost-effective, non-toxic, and environmentally friendly approach to obtaining nanoparticles. The biomolecules present in the plant extracts, such as phytochemicals, are responsible for the bioreduction and stabilization of the nanoparticles [72]. The studies suggest that metallic nanoparticles containing plant extracts have been used to treat bone disorders such as osteoporosis. The studies suggest that silver nanoparticles can inhibit differentiation into osteoclasts, indicating their potential as a treatment modality for bone-related diseases.

Besides morphology and adhesion changes, internalized phyto-nanoparticles can directly modulate intracellular signaling proteins and transcription cascades involved in differentiation. For instance, curcumin-gold nanoparticles were found to upregulate Ca2+/NFATc1 signaling through reactive oxygen species generation, consequently increasing alkaline phosphatase activity [73]. Resveratrol nanoparticles amplified miR-21 levels to suppress Smad-7 inhibitory effects on Runx2 and downstream effector activation leading to the commencement of osteoblastic gene expression programs [74]. In addition to osteoblastogenesis, a dynamic equilibrium between

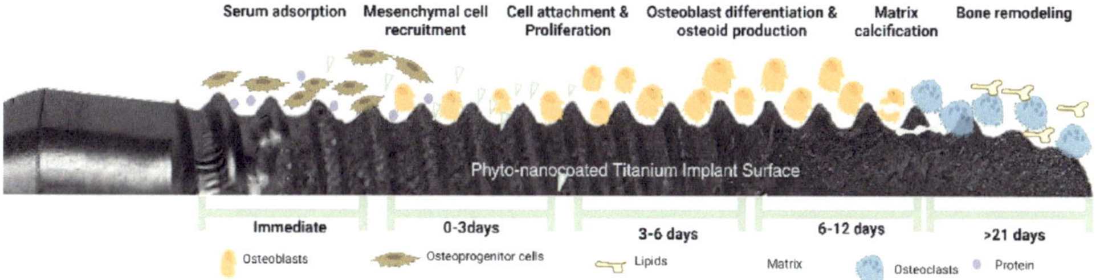

Figure 3.
Schematic representation of the cellular events occurring at the interface between a phyto-nanocoated implant and bone tissue during the healing process. The illustration depicts the key bone formation and remodeling stages, influenced by phyto-nanoparticles on the implant surface.

bone formation and resorption also necessitates the regulation of multinucleated osteoclasts from monocytic precursors. Undesirable excessive activity leads to net bone loss, compromising repair outcomes. As such, phyto-nanoparticles can target enhanced osteoblastogenesis with attenuated osteoclastogenesis [75]. Silica nanoparticles suppressed osteoclast differentiation and resorptive activity by downregulating NF-κB and interfering with RANK/RANKL signaling that initiates maturation. Meanwhile, hydroxyapatite nanoparticles mitigated reactive oxygen species propagation in osteoblasts subjected to oxidative challenge, preventing premature senescence and enabling sustained matrix deposition [76].

5.2 Drug delivery and sustained release

Plant nanoparticles are emerging as promising drug delivery systems and sustained-release vehicles because they can enhance therapeutic efficacy and mitigate side effects [77]. These nanoparticles, typically 10 to <1000 nm in size, can be engineered to encapsulate drugs and exhibit controlled release properties [78]. The physicochemical characteristics of nanoparticles, including size, surface area, surface chemistry, and shape, significantly impact their interactions within biological systems and are critical design parameters. For example, precise control over size and morphology is required to optimize performance and reduce toxicity. Furthermore, functionalizing the nanoparticle surface with polymers, antibodies, or other ligands facilitates active targeting of specific cells and tissues, thereby improving delivery capabilities [79].

Various nanoparticle platforms, such as lipid, polymer, and peptide nanoparticles, have been developed as drug delivery systems to transport therapeutic agents to intended sites within the body. These systems offer pharmacokinetic advantages compared to free drugs, enable targeting of specific cells, and mitigate off-target effects, thereby improving treatment efficacy [80]. The drug release kinetics can also be engineered by modifying nanoparticle size, surface traits, and composition to achieve sustained and controlled release profiles crucial for chronic therapies [81]. This targeted and sustained drug action reduces drug-induced toxicity while enhancing patient compliance through less frequent dosing regimens, ultimately translating to better patient outcomes. However, the clinical translation of plant nanoparticles warrants further research into the implications of their physicochemical attributes on biological interactions and the development of safe and efficacious drug delivery systems.

Phyto-nanoparticles act as versatile platforms for the intracellular delivery of osteogenic drugs to stimulate implanted scaffold cells or endogenous cells recruited to defect sites. Sustained release perpetuates bioactivity and enhances permeation throughout 3D-engineered tissues [82]. Nanoparticles facilitate passage through cell membranes for efficient internalization and residence within cytosol drug depots. Gradual diffusion or cumulative matrix erosion provides prolonged release kinetics that are optimal for maintaining cell stimulation without adverse effects from sudden bursts. Stimuli-responsive strategies using endogenous or exogenous triggers permit spatiotemporal control over release profiles [83]. Beyond growth factors, small molecule drugs have also been adapted into phyto-nanoparticles. Resveratrol-layered double hydroxide nanohybrids enabled tunable sustained release by diffusion control for over a month [84]. Rat calvarial defect treatment revealed up to 3-fold higher bone volumes than direct injection, confirming enhanced bioavailability and osteogenesis stimulation in vivo via the nanohybrid delivery system [85]. Curcumin nano-formulations similarly amplified therapeutic effects by increasing circulation half-life [86].

5.3 Anti-inflammatory and antimicrobial effects

Phyto-nanoparticles provide auxiliary anti-inflammatory and antimicrobial functionality alongside osteogenic stimulation effects to create optimal microenvironments facilitating repair [87]. Metabolically active compounds like polydatin and protocatechuic acid have been integrated into MSN mesoporous silica nanoparticles to dual-release anti-inflammatory osteogenic drugs [88]. Polydatin nanoparticles suppressed the secretion of inflammatory factors like TNF-α, IL-6, and nitric oxide in LPS-activated macrophages. The anti-inflammatory effects were further enhanced when co-delivered with bone morphogenetic protein two, stimulating mesenchymal stem cell recruitment and local regeneration. These synergistic combinations thus accelerate the resolution of inflammation to progress toward pro-osteogenic conditions [89]. Essential oils containing antimicrobial phytochemicals have been adapted onto osteoconductive bioceramic nanoparticles to combat bacterial infections [90]. Tea tree oil-functionalized magnesium phosphate nanoparticles provided a sustained release of antibacterial oil components alongside facilitating new bone growth [91]. The nanoparticles also induced minimal foreign body reaction and enhanced corrosion resistance compared to pure magnesium. These complementary osteogenic and antimicrobial properties will improve treatment outcomes for infected bone injuries [92].

Plant-mediated nanoparticles have significant anti-inflammatory and antimicrobial properties, making them promising candidates for biomedical applications. Specifically, silver and selenium nanoparticles synthesized using various plant extracts have shown potential as anti-inflammatory agents for treating conditions characterized by inflammation and antimicrobial agents for targeting resistant infections. Silver nanoparticles (AgNPs) synthesized using *Aloe vera*, green tea, grapefruit, *Mentha piperita*, and *Catharanthus roseus* extracts have exhibited anti-inflammatory capabilities [93, 94]. The anti-inflammatory effects make these AgNPs viable options for managing inflammatory ailments. Selenium nanoparticles (SeNPs) prepared using extracts of hawthorn fruit, onion, *Thymus vulgaris*, *Ceropegia bulbosa Roxb*, and *Diospyros Montana* have also demonstrated significant anti-inflammatory properties. These anti-inflammatory SeNPs hold promise as potential agents for treating inflammation-related diseases [95, 96]. Plant-mediated silver and selenium nanoparticles have also displayed broad-spectrum antimicrobial activity against various pathogenic bacteria and fungi. Their potent antimicrobial effects make these nanoparticles candidate alternatives to conventional antimicrobials for tackling drug-resistant infections. Plant-synthesized silver and selenium nanoparticles have shown considerable promise as anti-inflammatory agents for inflammatory diseases and antimicrobial agents for resistant infections [97]. Further research is warranted to translate these nanomaterials into clinical applications as anti-inflammatory and antimicrobial therapeutics.

6. Applications in bone regeneration

Capitalizing on their osteogenic stimulatory effects, phyto-nanoparticles have found widespread applications in designing advanced bone scaffolds, functionalizing orthopedic implants, and therapeutic carriers for bone disease treatments.

6.1 Scaffold materials for bone tissue engineering

Plant-derived nanoparticles are emerging as promising scaffold materials for bone tissue engineering owing to their biomimetic and osteoinductive properties. In particular, biocompatible silica nanoparticles from corn cob and rice husk stimulate osteoblast proliferation and bone growth while inhibiting osteoclasts, making them optimal scaffolds for bone disorders like osteoporosis [98, 99]. Beyond silica, calcium phosphate and gold nanoparticles also possess impressive osteogenic capabilities and have been studied as scaffolds for bone regeneration. For instance, strontium/magnesium-doped calcium phosphate nanoparticles have elicited positive in vitro responses from bone cells, underscoring their potential [100].

Capitalizing on the pro-osteogenic attributes, researchers have developed injectable hydrogels using composites of hydroxyapatite nanoparticles and plant derivatives like silk fibroin, cellulose, and chitosan [101]. Crosslinking chitosan-hydroxyapatite nanoparticles with aloe polysaccharides creates shear-thinning, self-recovery hydrogels suitable for minimally invasive delivery. The macroporous architecture enables bone marrow stem cell infiltration, proliferation, and osteogenic differentiation through controlled release of aloe bioactive phytochemicals, ultimately stimulating functional bone repair in vivo [102].

Plant nanocelluloses fabricated via acid hydrolysis of cellulose fibers also make highly porous bone scaffolds with mechanical integrity rivaling cancellous bones. The concomitant high-water retention facilitates nutrient diffusion and waste removal, enabling osteoblast migration and proliferation with early signs of matrix mineralization [103]. As the nanocelluloses degrade into non-toxic sugars, they mitigate long-term complications. Beyond direct bone formation, aloe polysaccharide nanoparticles delivering pro-angiogenic factors like VEGF from resident osteoblasts can also create vascularized grafts integrated with minimal fibrous scarring [46]. Such intelligently designed phyto-nanoparticles synchronize multiple mechanisms for synergistic bone regeneration.

6.2 Coatings for bone implants

Phyto-nanoparticles hold immense potential for surface modification of bone implants to enhance osseointegration. The current predominant use of bioinert metals like titanium often results in poor host tissue integration, provoking foreign body reactions, leading to fibrotic capsule formation, impairing implant-bone interlock, and providing infectious foci. Phyto-nanoparticle coatings present bioactive interfaces promoting bone cell migration and matrix deposition for accelerated anchorage [104]. Anti-inflammatory ingredients also mitigate immunogenic responses. Phyto-nanoparticle coatings aim to recapitulate multi-factorial extracellular niches by integrating osteoconductive, osteogenic, and anti-infective agents onto implant surfaces. For example, Sabir et al. fabricated zinc-doped hydroxyapatite silica coatings with clove extracts with innate antimicrobial properties. Sustained release of bioactive eugenol compounds inhibited adhesion and destroyed membranes of common pathogens, thus preventing implant-associated infections. The unimpeded growth of osteosarcoma cells also demonstrated excellent cytocompatibility [105].

Seeking dynamic interfaces, Motornov et al. [106] developed self-assembled films containing redox-responsive plant polyphenol nano-capsules on titanium dioxide nanotube arrays formed directly on titanium surfaces. The nano-capsules provided a controlled release of osteogenic and anti-inflammatory agents to stimulate endogenous cell activity. Redox triggers like hydrogen peroxide and ubiquitous glutathione unlocked cargo release by capsule swelling and membrane destabilization. Such innovative delivery systems enable spatiotemporal control, synchronizing therapeutic release profiles in tune with local biological cues [107].

Recent enthusiasm around graphene has sparked interest in phyto-mediated green synthesis of graphene-based implant coatings. Adding silver nanoparticles contributed to anti-infective effects against multidrug-resistant microbes. The accelerated hydroxyapatite deposition and alkaline phosphatase upregulation in osteoblasts cultured on these coatings demonstrated excellent biomineralization. Easy scalability makes such eco-friendly materials attractive for practical translational applications. Plant-derived nanoparticles can be used as coatings on dental and orthopedic implants to enhance their properties and performance. Zirconium nanoparticles from ginger and garlic have shown promise in enhancing dental implants' antimicrobial, mechanical, and osseointegration properties [108]. Silver nanoparticles from *Azadirachta indica* (Neem), *Aloe vera*, *Emblica Officinalis* (Amla), *Cinnamomum camphora* extract, and curcumin nanoparticles from turmeric have antimicrobial effects to reduce infections [53, 109–111]. Zinc oxide nanoparticles from Camellia sinensis have low cytotoxicity and biocompatibility as dental implant coatings [112]. Plant extracts like *Aloe vera*, green tea, and grapefruit have synthesized gold nanoparticles to improve implant biocompatibility, mechanical properties, antimicrobial activity, and osteoinduction [113].

6.3 Targeted therapy for bone diseases

Bone disorders like osteoporosis and infectious osteomyelitis remain challenging clinical issues as conventional treatments struggle to stimulate regeneration and penetrate dense mineralized matrices. Phyto-nanoparticles present innovative solutions for targeted drug delivery to diseased skeletal sites by protecting cargo drugs from bodily clearance and providing sustained release. Their nanoscale size facilitates extravasation through porous vasculatures nourishing skeletal tissues. Concurrent multimodal imaging enables tracking to verify localization. Seeking osteo-targetability, Liang et al. [114] prepared calcium-deficient hydroxyapatite nanoparticles with high binding affinity to the bone matrix. Covalent tethering of the anti-osteoporotic bisphosphonate alendronate further augmented hydroxyapatite specificity for skeleton tissues. Phyto-sourced berberine alkaloids with anti-osteoporotic effects were then loaded into the nanoparticles. Selective in vivo depot within bone enabled sustained berberine release, stimulating osteoblast differentiation while ameliorating ovariectomy-induced bone loss [112]. Such targeted delivery maximizes therapeutic indexes at diseased sites while avoiding systemic exposure.

Contending with osteomyelitis, Alegrete et al. [115] devised starch-based nanocarriers for bone-selective delivery of vancomycin antibiotics. Cationic surface coatings enabled electrostatic loading of anionic vancomycin molecules with 85% efficiency. Sustained vancomycin release inhibited bacterial growth for a week, reducing inflammatory TNF-alpha and osteoclast activity. Osteoblast proliferation also recovered. Effective infection control coupled with mitigated bone damage illustrates the merits of phyto-nanoparticles for therapeutic delivery, combining innate bioactivity and biocompatibility [113]. In summary, these regenerative medicine niches spanning tissue engineering, implant modification, and drug delivery vehicles provide promising clinical translation pathways capitalizing on emergent phyto-nanotechnology research. A common theme is the recognition of how multifaceted extracellular milieu factors synergistically direct tissue healing outcomes. Appropriately designed phyto-nanoparticles offer intelligently engineered tools integrating biological and physical inputs to stimulate endogenous regenerative responses.

7. Future perspectives and conclusions

Phyto-nanotechnology remains in its early stages, with further innovations in fabrication strategies and biomedical applications necessary to fully tap this vast, untapped potential. Ongoing adoption of personalized medicine approaches appears highly feasible. Additionally, hybrid platforms synergistically combining plant nanoparticles with complementary nanostructures and technologies could engender augmented therapeutic capacities exceeding individual components. In summary, these promising directions forecast next-generation phyto-nanosystems dramatically advancing bone regenerative capabilities and transforming clinical practice. Research fusing plant-based nanomaterials with technologies like 3D bioprinting and externally triggered smart nanoparticles could enable customized patient therapies and enhanced control over healing outcomes. Further research and development focusing on efficacy, safety, and clinical integration will be vital to realizing the full clinical potential of these powerful emerging approaches.

7.1 Innovations in synthesis and application

In recent years, the integration and use of plant-sourced nanoparticles in medicine and dentistry have gained considerable interest. Adopting plant extracts to generate nanoparticles provides multiple benefits over traditional approaches, including cost-effectiveness, environmental sustainability, and control over nanoparticle structure. This method also overcomes nanoparticle clustering during formation, enabling the production of diverse nanoparticle types. Plant-based nanoparticles have shown promise in improving dental implants' compatibility, durability, and antibacterial properties. Creating bone-targeted nanoparticles and carriers from plants also holds the potential for enhancing osteoporosis treatment by improving drug delivery, minimizing side effects, and boosting the efficacy and safety of osteoporosis medications. The future outlook of plant nanoparticles is promising, with ongoing research on developing new synthesis techniques, characterization methods, and applications. Plant nanoparticles offer advantages over conventional physicochemical preparations, including cost-effectiveness, eco-friendliness, morphology control, and the ability to prevent nanoparticle agglomeration during production for a wide range of nanoparticles.

7.2 Integration with other nanotechnologies

Integrating plant-sourced nanoparticles with other nanostructures, materials, and technologies shows immense potential for synergistic platforms that enhance efficacy beyond individual components. Hybrid nanocomposites combining cellulose, silk, or chitosan phyto-nanoparticles with osteoconductive hydroxyapatites or bioactive glasses can produce scaffolds that mimic complementary aspects of native bone extracellular matrix. This could provide more biomimetic environments to guide bone formation. Incorporating magnetic and plasmonic metal nanoparticles within phyto-nanoparticle matrices could enable external manipulation and stimulation using alternating magnetic fields and laser irradiation. This may allow spatiotemporal control over scaffold activities to better direct cell differentiation and healing. Imaging techniques like surface-enhanced Raman spectroscopy using phyto-reduced gold nanorods also facilitate deeper tracking of bone regeneration in vivo, which is crucial for evaluating translation potential.

Bridging niche applications, fluoride-releasing phyto-nanoparticles could have concurrent antibacterial effects against cariogenic pathogens responsible for dental caries and infections that endanger orthopedic implants. Phyto-nanosystems may also help mitigate bone loss side effects of anticancer medications. Beyond passive carriers, cell membrane-coated phyto-nanoparticles cloaked with blood cell or stem cell membranes may enable biomimetic vehicles for immune system evasion and enhanced tissue penetration. These multifunctional capacities gained from hybridization with emerging nanotechnologies promise innovative solutions for enhanced bone repair. In summary, further research at the intersection of plant biosciences and nanotechnology can realize smarter phyto-nanomaterials designed to synchronize the complex extracellular signals that collectively coordinate optimal healing. Seamless integration into clinical practice promises transformative positive impacts on restoring skeletal function for countless worldwide suffering from bone diseases or injuries.

7.3 Potential in personalized medicine

Inter-patient variability and unique defect microenvironments contribute to inconsistent outcomes using standardized treatments. Transitioning toward personalized medicine paradigms that tailor therapies to individual needs could address these inconsistencies. Readily functionalized phyto-nanoparticles with tunable properties present versatile platforms that enable patient-specific formulations. Nuclear imaging and magnetic relaxation switching may non-invasively track nanoparticle pharmacokinetics and localization within distinct wound sites. This facilitates identifying disease subsets most responsive to particular formulations. Omics profiling discerns proteomic biomarkers and implicated genetic polymorphisms guiding formulation optimization, including specific phytochemical agents targeting dysregulated pathways. Patient-derived cells could determine optimal scaffolded cargo combinations (e.g., cells, genes, drugs) for improved engraftment. 3D bioprinting also enables designing custom macro-architecture and internal porous features adapted to scanned defect volumes. On-demand activation of smart phyto-nanomaterials with external triggers (ultrasound, electromagnetic fields) further permits unprecedented spatiotemporal control over particular cellular stimulation events. These could be programmed in response to personalized healing events like inflammation resolution or cell mobilization waves. Such dynamic, personalized therapies will ultimately improve the consistency and quality of treatment outcomes.

Conflict of interest

The authors declare no conflict of interest.

Author details

Nandita Suresh[1*], Betsy Joseph[1,2], Tuomas Waltimo[3] and Sukumaran Anil[4,5]

1 Department of Oral and Maxillofacial Diseases, Helsinki University and University Hospital, Helsinki, Finland

2 Department of Periodontics, Saveetha Dental College and Hospitals, Saveetha Institute of Medical and Technical Sciences, Chennai, India

3 Department of Oral Health and Medicine, University Center for Dental Medicine Basel, University of Basel, Basel, Switzerland

4 Department of Dentistry, Hamad Medical Corporation, Doha, Qatar

5 College of Dental Medicine, Qatar University, Doha, Qatar

*Address all correspondence to: dr.nanditasuresh@gmail.com

References

[1] Bayda S, Adeel M, Tuccinardi T, Cordani M, Rizzolio F. The history of nanoscience and nanotechnology: From chemical-physical applications to nanomedicine. Molecules. 2019;**25**:1-15. Epub 20191227. DOI: 10.3390/molecules25010112

[2] Malik S, Muhammad K, Waheed Y. Emerging applications of nanotechnology in healthcare and medicine. Molecules. 2023;**28**:1-30. Epub 20230914. DOI: 10.3390/molecules28186624

[3] Amini AR, Laurencin CT, Nukavarapu SP. Bone tissue engineering: Recent advances and challenges. Critical Reviews in Biomedical Engineering. 2012;**40**:363-408. DOI: 10.1615/critrevbiomedeng.v40.i5.10

[4] Hong MH, Lee JH, Jung HS, Shin H, Shin H. Biomineralization of bone tissue: Calcium phosphate-based inorganics in collagen fibrillar organic matrices. Biomaterials Research. 2022;**26**:42. Epub 20220906. DOI: 10.1186/s40824-022-00288-0

[5] Jiang S, Wang M, He J. A review of biomimetic scaffolds for bone regeneration: Toward a cell-free strategy. Bioengineering & Translational Medicine. 2021;**6**:e10206. Epub 20201215. DOI: 10.1002/btm2.10206

[6] Hasan A, Morshed M, Memic A, Hassan S, Webster TJ, Marei HE. Nanoparticles in tissue engineering: Applications, challenges and prospects. International Journal of Nanomedicine. 2018;**13**:5637-5655. Epub 20180924. DOI: 10.2147/IJN.S153758

[7] Mahmoud NS, Ahmed HH, Mohamed MR, Amr KS, Aglan HA, Ali MAM, et al. Role of nanoparticles in osteogenic differentiation of bone marrow mesenchymal stem cells. Cytotechnology. 2020;**72**:1-22. Epub 20191113. DOI: 10.1007/s10616-019-00353-y

[8] Udomluck N, Koh WG, Lim DJ, Park H. Recent developments in nanofiber fabrication and modification for bone tissue engineering. International Journal of Molecular Sciences. 2019;**21**:1-16. Epub 20191221. DOI: 10.3390/ijms21010099

[9] Hano C, Abbasi BH. Plant-based green synthesis of nanoparticles: Production, characterization and applications. Biomolecules. 2021;**12**:1-9. Epub 20211225. DOI: 10.3390/biom12010031

[10] Lee J, Park EY, Lee J. Non-toxic nanoparticles from phytochemicals: Preparation and biomedical application. Bioprocess and Biosystems Engineering. 2014;**37**:983-989. Epub 20131122 10.1007/s00449-013-1091-3

[11] Husen A, Siddiqi KS. Phytosynthesis of nanoparticles: Concept, controversy and application. Nanoscale Research Letters. 2014;**9**:229. Epub 20140512. DOI: 10.1186/1556-276X-9-229

[12] Jadhav K, Hr R, Deshpande S, Jagwani S, Dhamecha D, Jalalpure S, et al. Phytosynthesis of gold nanoparticles: Characterization, biocompatibility, and evaluation of its osteoinductive potential for application in implant dentistry. Materials Science & Engineering. C, Materials for Biological Applications. 2018;**93**:664-670. Epub 20180810. DOI: 10.1016/j.msec.2018.08.028

[13] Tiwari S, Verma SK, Bhagat P, Yadav S, Sharma R, Aseri GK, et al. An

overview of the phytosynthesis of various metal nanoparticles. 3 Biotech. 2021;**11**:478. Epub 20211029. DOI: 10.1007/s13205-021-03014-0

[14] Yao Q, Yuan X, Fung V, Yu Y, Leong DT, Jiang DE, et al. Understanding seed-mediated growth of gold nanoclusters at molecular level. Nature Communications. 2017;**8**:927. Epub 20171013. DOI: 10.1038/s41467-017-00970-1

[15] Ashraf H, Anjum T, Riaz S, Naseem S. Microwave-assisted green synthesis and characterization of silver nanoparticles using Melia azedarach for the management of fusarium wilt in tomato. Frontiers in Microbiology. 2020;**11**:238. Epub 20200310. DOI: 10.3389/fmicb.2020.00238

[16] Gao L, Mei S, Ma H, Chen X. Ultrasound-assisted green synthesis of gold nanoparticles using citrus peel extract and their enhanced anti-inflammatory activity. Ultrasonics Sonochemistry. 2022;**83**:105940. Epub 20220203. DOI: 10.1016/j.ultsonch.2022.105940

[17] Bhilkar PR, Bodhne AS, Yerpude ST, Madankar RS, Somkuwar SR, Daddemal-Chaudhary AR, et al. Phyto-derived metal nanoparticles: Prominent tool for biomedical applications. OpenNano. 2023;**14**:100192. DOI: 10.1016/j.onano.2023.100192

[18] Puri A, Patil S, Mulik M. Biomedical applications of biogenic phytonanoparticles a review. International Journal of Botany. 2021;**6**:534-540

[19] Thatyana M, Dube NP, Kemboi D, Manicum AE, Mokgalaka-Fleischmann NS, Tembu JV. Advances in phytonanotechnology: A plant-mediated green synthesis of metal nanoparticles using phyllanthus plant extracts and their antimicrobial and anticancer applications. Nanomaterials (Basel). 2023;**13**:1-30. Epub 20230922. DOI: 10.3390/nano13192616

[20] Yusuf A, Almotairy ARZ, Henidi H, Alshehri OY, Aldughaim MS. Nanoparticles as drug delivery systems: A review of the implication of nanoparticles' physicochemical properties on responses in biological systems. Polymers (Basel). 2023;**15**:1-26. Epub 20230323. DOI: 10.3390/polym15071596

[21] Hafez, Ghoran S, Calcaterra A, Abbasi M, Taktaz F, Nieselt K, Babaei E. Curcumin-based nanoformulations: A promising adjuvant towards cancer treatment. Molecules. 2022;**27**:1-29. Epub 20220816. DOI: 10.3390/molecules27165236

[22] Kazemi S, Hosseingholian A, Gohari SD, Feirahi F, Moammeri F, Mesbahian G, et al. Recent advances in green synthesized nanoparticles: From production to application. Materials Today Sustainability. 2023;**24**:100500. DOI: 10.1016/j.mtsust.2023.100500

[23] Hajialyani M, Tewari D, Sobarzo-Sánchez E, Nabavi SM, Farzaei MH, Abdollahi M. Natural product-based nanomedicines for wound healing purposes: Therapeutic targets and drug delivery systems. International Journal of Nanomedicine. 2018;**13**:5023-5043. Epub 20180903. DOI: 10.2147/ijn.S174072

[24] Abuzeid HM, Julien CM, Zhu L, Hashem AM. Green synthesis of nanoparticles and their energy storage. Environmental, and Biomedical Applications Crystals. 2023;**13**:1576. DOI: 10.3390/cryst13111576

[25] Adeyemi JO, Oriola AO, Onwudiwe DC, Oyedeji AO. Plant

extracts mediated metal-based nanoparticles: Synthesis and biological applications. Biomolecules. 2022;**12**:1-28. Epub 20220424. DOI: 10.3390/biom12050627

[26] Mehan S, Arora N, Bhalla S, Khan A, Rehman MU, Alghamdi BS, et al. Involvement of phytochemical-encapsulated nanoparticles' interaction with cellular signalling in the amelioration of benign and malignant brain tumours. Molecules. 2022;**27**:1-27. Epub 20220601. DOI: 10.3390/molecules27113561

[27] Vohra K, Dureja H, Garg V, Dutt R. Current trends in phyto-cancer therapy using nanoparticles current. Nanomedicine. 2019;**9**:30-45. DOI: 10.2174/2468187308666180613102448

[28] Singh H, Desimone MF, Pandya S, Jasani S, George N, Adnan M, et al. Revisiting the green synthesis of nanoparticles: Uncovering influences of plant extracts as reducing agents for enhanced synthesis efficiency and its biomedical applications. International Journal of Nanomedicine. 2023;**18**:4727-4750. Epub 20230818. DOI: 10.2147/ijn.S419369

[29] Osman AI, Zhang Y, Farghali M, Rashwan AK, Eltaweil AS, Abd El-Monaem EM, et al. Synthesis of green nanoparticles for energy, biomedical, environmental, agricultural, and food applications: A review. Environmental Chemistry Letters. 2024;**22**:841-887. DOI: 10.1007/s10311-023-01682-3

[30] Sharma R, Sharma N, Prashar A, Hansa A, Asgari Lajayer B, Price GW. Unraveling the plethora of toxicological implications of nanoparticles on living organisms and recent insights into different remediation strategies: A comprehensive review. Science of the Total Environment. 2024;**906**:167697. DOI: 10.1016/j.scitotenv.2023.167697

[31] Ezike TC, Okpala US, Onoja UL, Nwike CP, Ezeako EC, Okpara OJ, et al. Advances in drug delivery systems, challenges and future directions. Heliyon. 2023;**9**:e17488. Epub 20230624. DOI: 10.1016/j.heliyon.2023.e17488

[32] Mohammadinejad R, Karimi S, Iravani S, Varma RS. Plant-derived nanostructures: Types and applications. Green Chemistry. 2016;**18**:20-52. DOI: 10.1039/c5gc01403d

[33] Gopal J, Muthu M, Paul D, Kim DH, Chun S. Bactericidal activity of green tea extracts: The importance of catechin containing nano particles. Scientific Reports. 2016;**6**:19710. Epub 20160128. DOI: 10.1038/srep19710

[34] Polito CA, Cai ZY, Shi YL, Li XM, Yang R, Shi M, et al. Association of tea consumption with risk of Alzheimer's disease and anti-beta-amyloid effects of tea. Nutrients. 2018;**10**:1-18. Epub 20180522. DOI: 10.3390/nu10050655

[35] Kim HM, Kim J. The effects of green tea on obesity and type 2 diabetes. Diabetes & Metabolism Journal. 2013;**37**:173-175. DOI: 10.4093/dmj.2013.37.3.173

[36] Ninsiima HI, Eze ED, Ssekatawa K, Nalugo H, Asekenye C, Onanyang D, et al. Green tea silver nanoparticles improve physiological motor and cognitive function in BALB/c mice during inflammation. Heliyon. 2023;**9**:e13922. Epub 20230221. DOI: 10.1016/j.heliyon.2023.e13922

[37] Lin SY, Kan JY, Lu CC, Huang HH, Cheng TL, Huang HT, et al. Green tea catechin (−)-epigallocatechin-3-gallate (EGCG) facilitates fracture healing.

Biomolecules. 2020;**10**:1-10. Epub 20200416. DOI: 10.3390/biom10040620

[38] Shen CL, Yeh JK, Cao JJ, Wang JS. Green tea and bone metabolism. Nutrition Research. 2009;**29**:437-456. DOI: 10.1016/j.nutres.2009.06.008

[39] Chu C, Deng J, Man Y, Qu Y. Green tea extracts epigallocatechin-3-gallate for different treatments. BioMed Research International. 2017;**2017**:5615647. Epub 20170813. DOI: 10.1155/2017/5615647

[40] Zhang X, He J, Qiao L, Wang Z, Zheng Q, Xiong C, et al. 3D printed PCLA scaffold with nano-hydroxyapatite coating doped green tea EGCG promotes bone growth and inhibits multidrug-resistant bacteria colonization. Cell Proliferation. 2022;**55**:e13289. Epub 20220705. DOI: 10.1111/cpr.13289

[41] Huang HT, Cheng TL, Lin SY, Ho CJ, Chyu JY, Yang RS, et al. Osteoprotective roles of green tea catechins. Antioxidants (Basel). 2020;**9**:1136. Epub 20201116. DOI: 10.3390/antiox9111136

[42] Sanchez M, Gonzalez-Burgos E, Iglesias I, Gomez-Serranillos MP. Pharmacological update properties of aloe vera and its major active constituents. Molecules. 2020;**25**:1-37. Epub 20200313. DOI: 10.3390/molecules25061324

[43] Pradeep AR, Garg V, Raju A, Singh P. Adjunctive local delivery of aloe vera gel in patients with type 2 diabetes and chronic periodontitis: A randomized, controlled clinical trial. Journal of Periodontology. 2016;**87**:268-274. Epub 20151008. DOI: 10.1902/jop.2015.150161

[44] Alinejad-Mofrad S, Foadoddini M, Saadatjoo SA, Shayesteh M. Improvement of glucose and lipid profile status with aloe vera in pre-diabetic subjects: A randomized controlled-trial. Journal of Diabetes and Metabolic Disorders. 2015;**14**:22. Epub 20150409. DOI: 10.1186/s40200-015-0137-2

[45] Teplicki E, Ma Q, Castillo DE, Zarei M, Hustad AP, Chen J, et al. The effects of aloe vera on wound healing in cell proliferation, migration, and viability. Wounds. 2018;**30**:263-268

[46] Yao XW, Liu HD, Ren MX, Li TL, Jiang WK, Zhou Z, et al. Aloe polysaccharide promotes osteogenesis potential of adipose-derived stromal cells via BMP-2/Smads and prevents ovariectomized-induced osteoporosis. Molecular Biology Reports. 2022;**49**:11913-11924. Epub 20221015. DOI: 10.1007/s11033-022-08003-x

[47] Banerjee D, Bose S. Effects of aloe vera gel extract in doped hydroxyapatite-coated titanium implants on in vivo and in vitro biological properties. ACS Applied Bio Materials. 2019;**2**:3194-3202. Epub 20190719. DOI: 10.1021/acsabm.9b00077

[48] Ghorbani M, Nezhad-Mokhtari P, Ramazani S. Aloe vera-loaded nanofibrous scaffold based on zein/polycaprolactone/collagen for wound healing. International Journal of Biological Macromolecules. 2020;**153**:921-930. Epub 20200306. DOI: 10.1016/j.ijbiomac.2020.03.036

[49] Prasad S, Tyagi AK, Aggarwal BB. Recent developments in delivery, bioavailability, absorption and metabolism of curcumin: The golden pigment from golden spice. Cancer Research and Treatment. 2014;**46**:2-18. Epub 20140115. DOI: 10.4143/crt.2014.46.1.2

[50] Ma Z, Wang N, He H, Tang X. Pharmaceutical strategies of improving oral systemic bioavailability of curcumin for clinical application. Journal of

Controlled Release. 2019;**316**:359-380. Epub 20191102. DOI: 10.1016/j.jconrel.2019.10.053

[51] Srinivasan K. Black pepper and its pungent principle-piperine: A review of diverse physiological effects. Critical Reviews in Food Science and Nutrition. 2007;**47**:735-748. DOI: 10.1080/10408390601062054

[52] Punfa W, Yodkeeree S, Pitchakarn P, Ampasavate C, Limtrakul P. Enhancement of cellular uptake and cytotoxicity of curcumin-loaded PLGA nanoparticles by conjugation with anti-P-glycoprotein in drug resistance cancer cells. Acta Pharmacologica Sinica. 2012;**33**:823-831. Epub 20120514. DOI: 10.1038/aps.2012.34

[53] Bhawana I, Basniwal RK, Buttar HS, Jain VK, Jain N. Curcumin nanoparticles: Preparation, characterization, and antimicrobial study. Journal of Agricultural and Food Chemistry. 2011. Epub 20110215;**59**:2056-2061. DOI: 10.1021/jf104402t

[54] Ubeyitogullari A, Ciftci ON. A novel and green nanoparticle formation approach to forming low-crystallinity curcumin nanoparticles to improve curcumin's bioaccessibility. Scientific Reports. 2019;**9**:19112. Epub 20191213. DOI: 10.1038/s41598-019-55619-4

[55] Rahimi HR, Nedaeinia R, Sepehri Shamloo A, Nikdoust S, Kazemi OR. Novel delivery system for natural products: Nano-curcumin formulations. Avicenna Journal of Phytomedicine. 2016;**6**:383-398

[56] Maleki Dizaj S, Shokrgozar H, Yazdani J, Memar MY, Sharifi S, Ghavimi MA. Antibacterial effects of curcumin nanocrystals against porphyromonas gingivalis isolated from patients with implant failure. Clinics and Practice. 2022;**12**:809-817. Epub 20221006. DOI: 10.3390/clinpract12050085

[57] Al-Ani LA, Kadir FA, Hashim NM, Julkapli NM, Seyfoddin A, Lu J, et al. The impact of curcumin-graphene based nanoformulation on cellular interaction and redox-activated apoptosis: An in vitro colon cancer study. Heliyon. 2020;**6**:e05360. Epub 20201102. DOI: 10.1016/j.heliyon.2020.e05360

[58] Gan J, Deng X, Le Y, Lai J, Liao X. The development of naringin for use against bone and cartilage disorders. Molecules. 2023;**28**:1-20. Epub 20230425. DOI: 10.3390/molecules28093716

[59] Fan J, Li J, Fan Q. Naringin promotes differentiation of bone marrow stem cells into osteoblasts by upregulating the expression levels of microRNA-20a and downregulating the expression levels of PPARgamma. Molecular Medicine Reports. 2015;**12**:4759-4765. Epub 20150624. DOI: 10.3892/mmr.2015.3996

[60] Heo JS, Lee SG, Kim HO. The flavonoid glabridin induces OCT4 to enhance osteogenetic potential in mesenchymal stem cells. Stem Cells International. 2017;**2017**:6921703. Epub 20171114. DOI: 10.1155/2017/6921703

[61] Al-Anazi AF, Qureshi VF, Javaid K, Qureshi S. Preventive effects of phytoestrogens against postmenopausal osteoporosis as compared to the available therapeutic choices: An overview. Journal of Natural Science, Biology, and Medicine. 2011;**2**:154-163. DOI: 10.4103/0976-9668.92322

[62] Yang J, Zhang L, Ding Q, Zhang S, Sun S, Liu W, et al. Flavonoid-loaded biomaterials in bone defect repair. Molecules. 2023;**28**:6888. Epub 20230930. DOI: 10.3390/molecules28196888

[63] Wong SK, Chin KY, Ima-Nirwana S. Quercetin as an agent for protecting the bone: A review of the current evidence. International Journal of Molecular Sciences. 2020;**21**:1-37. Epub 20200903. DOI: 10.3390/ijms21176448

[64] Szwed-Georgiou A, Plocinski P, Kupikowska-Stobba B, Urbaniak MM, Rusek-Wala P, Szustakiewicz K, et al. Bioactive materials for bone regeneration: Biomolecules and delivery systems. ACS Biomaterials Science & Engineering. 2023;**9**:5222-5254. Epub 20230816. DOI: 10.1021/acsbiomaterials.3c00609

[65] Kim JL, Park SH, Jeong D, Nam JS, Kang YH. Osteogenic activity of silymarin through enhancement of alkaline phosphatase and osteocalcin in osteoblasts and tibia-fractured mice. Experimental Biology and Medicine (Maywood, N.J.). 2012;**237**:417-428. Epub 20120410. DOI: 10.1258/ebm.2011.011376

[66] Ratan ZA, Haidere MF, Hong YH, Park SH, Lee JO, Lee J, et al. Pharmacological potential of ginseng and its major component ginsenosides. Journal of Ginseng Research. 2021;**45**:199-210. Epub 20200325. DOI: 10.1016/j.jgr.2020.02.004

[67] Gupta A, Mehta SK, Kumar A, Singh S. Advent of phytobiologics and nano-interventions for bone remodeling: A comprehensive review. Critical Reviews in Biotechnology. 2023;**43**:142-169. Epub 20211226. DOI: 10.1080/07388551.2021.2010031

[68] Gao W, Liang C, Zhao K, Hou M, Wen Y. Multifunctional gold nanoparticles for osteoporosis: Synthesis, mechanism and therapeutic applications. Journal of Translational Medicine. 2023;**21**:889. Epub 20231207. DOI: 10.1186/s12967-023-04594-6

[69] Luo J, Walker M, Xiao Y, Donnelly H, Dalby MJ, Salmeron-Sanchez M. The influence of nanotopography on cell behaviour through interactions with the extracellular matrix - A review. Bioactive Materials. 2022;**15**:145-159. Epub 20211221. DOI: 10.1016/j.bioactmat.2021.11.024

[70] Wutticharoenmongkol P, Pavasant P, Supaphol P. Osteoblastic phenotype expression of MC3T3-E1 cultured on electrospun polycaprolactone fiber mats filled with hydroxyapatite nanoparticles. Biomacromolecules. 2007;**8**:2602-2610. Epub 20070727. DOI: 10.1021/bm700451p

[71] Marycz K, Sobierajska P, Roecken M, Kornicka-Garbowska K, Kepska M, Idczak R, et al. Iron oxides nanoparticles (IOs) exposed to magnetic field promote expression of osteogenic markers in osteoblasts through integrin alpha-3 (INTa-3) activation, inhibits osteoclasts activity and exerts anti-inflammatory action. Journal of Nanobiotechnology. 2020;**18**:33. Epub 20200218. DOI: 10.1186/s12951-020-00590-w

[72] Saif S, Tahir A, Chen Y. Green synthesis of iron nanoparticles and their environmental applications and implications. Nanomaterials (Basel). 2016;**6**:1-26. Epub 20161112. DOI: 10.3390/nano6110209

[73] Chopra H, Dey PS, Das D, Bhattacharya T, Shah M, Mubin S, et al. Curcumin nanoparticles as promising therapeutic agents for drug targets. Molecules. 2021;**26**:1-28. Epub 20210818. DOI: 10.3390/molecules26164998

[74] Wang J, He F, Chen L, Li Q, Jin S, Zheng H, et al. Resveratrol inhibits pulmonary fibrosis by regulating miR-21 through MAPK/AP-1 pathways. Biomedicine & Pharmacotherapy. 2018;**105**:37-44. Epub 20180526. DOI: 10.1016/j.biopha.2018.05.104

[75] Liu K, Wang Z, Liu J, Zhao W, Qiao F, He Q, et al. Atsttrin regulates osteoblastogenesis and osteoclastogenesis through the TNFR pathway. Communications Biology. 2023;**6**:1251. Epub 20231211. DOI: 10.1038/s42003-023-05635-y

[76] Yin Z, Gong G, Liu X, Yin J. Mechanism of regulating macrophages/osteoclasts in attenuating wear particle-induced aseptic osteolysis. Frontiers in Immunology. 2023;**14**:1274679. Epub 20231004. DOI: 10.3389/fimmu.2023.1274679

[77] Patra JK, Das G, Fraceto LF, Campos EVR, Rodriguez-Torres MDP, Acosta-Torres LS, et al. Nano based drug delivery systems: Recent developments and future prospects. Journal of Nanobiotechnology. 2018;**16**:71. Epub 20180919. DOI: 10.1186/s12951-018-0392-8

[78] Mudshinge SR, Deore AB, Patil S, Bhalgat CM. Nanoparticles: Emerging carriers for drug delivery. Saudi Pharmaceutical Journal. 2011;**19**:129-141. Epub 20110421. DOI: 10.1016/j.jsps.2011.04.001

[79] Yagublu V, Karimova A, Hajibabazadeh J, Reissfelder C, Muradov M, Bellucci S, et al. Overview of physicochemical properties of nanoparticles as drug carriers for targeted cancer therapy. Journal of Functional Biomaterials. 2022;**13**:1-11. Epub 20221020. DOI: 10.3390/jfb13040196

[80] Sarvarian P, Samadi P, Gholipour E, Shams Asenjan K, Hojjat-Farsangi M, Motavalli R, et al. Application of emerging plant-derived nanoparticles as a novel approach for nano-drug delivery systems. Immunological Investigations. 2022;**51**:1039-1059. Epub 20210225. DOI: 10.1080/08820139.2021.1891094

[81] Rizvi SAA, Saleh AM. Applications of nanoparticle systems in drug delivery technology. Saudi Pharmaceutical Journal. 2018;**26**:64-70. Epub 20171025. DOI: 10.1016/j.jsps.2017.10.012

[82] Wen J, Cai D, Gao W, He R, Li Y, Zhou Y, et al. Osteoimmunomodulatory nanoparticles for bone regeneration. Nanomaterials (Basel). 2023;**13**:1-21. Epub 20230210. DOI: 10.3390/nano13040692

[83] Wen J, Li H, Dai H, Hua S, Long X, Li H, et al. Intra-articular nanoparticles based therapies for osteoarthritis and rheumatoid arthritis management. Materials Today Bio. 2023;**19**:100597. Epub 20230226. DOI: 10.1016/j.mtbio.2023.100597

[84] Herrera-Arozamena C, Estrada-Valencia M, Lopez-Caballero P, Perez C, Morales-Garcia JA, Perez-Castillo A, et al. Resveratrol-based MTDLs to stimulate defensive and regenerative pathways and block early events in neurodegenerative cascades. Journal of Medicinal Chemistry. 2022;**65**:4727-4751. Epub 20220304. DOI: 10.1021/acs.jmedchem.1c01883

[85] Stephan SJ, Tholpady SS, Gross B, Petrie-Aronin CE, Botchway EA, Nair LS, et al. Injectable tissue-engineered bone repair of a rat calvarial defect. Laryngoscope. 2010;**120**:895-901. DOI: 10.1002/lary.20624

[86] Tagde P, Tagde P, Islam F, Tagde S, Shah M, Hussain ZD, et al. The multifaceted role of curcumin in advanced nanocurcumin form in the treatment and management of chronic disorders. Molecules. 2021;**26**:1-33. Epub 20211124. DOI: 10.3390/molecules26237109

[87] Nandhini SN, Sisubalan N, Vijayan A, Karthikeyan C, Gnanaraj M,

Gideon DAM, et al. Recent advances in green synthesized nanoparticles for bactericidal and wound healing applications. Heliyon. 2023;**9**:e13128. Epub 20230121. DOI: 10.1016/j.heliyon.2023.e13128

[88] Sandomierski M, Chojnacka M, Dlugosz M, Pokora M, Zwolinska J, Majchrzycki L, et al. Mesoporous silica modified with polydopamine and zinc ions as a potential carrier in the controlled release of mercaptopurine. Materials (Basel). 2023;**16**:1-16. Epub 20230613. DOI: 10.3390/ma16124358

[89] Li W, Xiang Z, Yu W, Huang X, Jiang Q, Abumansour A, et al. Natural compounds and mesenchymal stem cells: Implications for inflammatory-impaired tissue regeneration. Stem Cell Research & Therapy. 2024;**15**:34. Epub 20240207. DOI: 10.1186/s13287-024-03641-3

[90] Ghosh S, Nandi S, Basu T. Nano-antibacterials using medicinal plant components: An overview. Frontiers in Microbiology. 2021;**12**:768739. Epub 20220222. DOI: 10.3389/fmicb.2021.768739

[91] Manzanelli FA, Ravetti S, Brignone SG, Garro AG, Martinez SR, Vallejo MG, et al. Enhancing the functional properties of tea tree oil: In vitro antimicrobial activity and microencapsulation strategy. Pharmaceutics. 2023;**15**:1-17. Epub 20231019. DOI: 10.3390/pharmaceutics15102489

[92] Zhong X, Gao F, Wei H, Zhou H, Zhou X. Functionalization of mesoporous silica as an effective composite carrier for essential oils with improved sustained release behavior and long-term antibacterial performance. Nanotechnology. 2021;**33**:035706. Epub 20211029. DOI: 10.1088/1361-6528/ac2fe2

[93] Mustapha T, Misni N, Ithnin NR, Daskum AM, Unyah NZ. A review on plants and microorganisms mediated synthesis of silver nanoparticles, role of plants metabolites and applications. International Journal of Environmental Research and Public Health. 2022;**19**:1-17. Epub 20220107. DOI: 10.3390/ijerph19020674

[94] Ahmed S, Ahmad M, Swami BL, Ikram S. A review on plants extract mediated synthesis of silver nanoparticles for antimicrobial applications: A green expertise. Journal of Advanced Research. 2016;**7**:17-28. Epub 20150309. DOI: 10.1016/j.jare.2015.02.007

[95] Pyrzynska K, Sentkowska A. Biosynthesis of selenium nanoparticles using plant extracts. Journal of Nanostructure in Chemistry. 2021;**12**:467-480. DOI: 10.1007/s40097-021-00435-4

[96] Pandiyan I, Sri SD, Indiran MA, Rathinavelu PK, Prabakar J, Rajeshkumar S. Antioxidant, anti-inflammatory activity of Thymus vulgaris-mediated selenium nanoparticles: An in vitro study. Journal of Conservative Dentistry. 2022;**25**:241-245. Epub 20220613. DOI: 10.4103/JCD.JCD_369_21

[97] Sans-Serramitjana E, Obreque M, Munoz F, Zaror C, Mora ML, Vinas M, et al. Antimicrobial activity of selenium nanoparticles (SeNPs) against potentially pathogenic oral microorganisms: A scoping review. Pharmaceutics. 2023;**15**:1-22. Epub 20230831. DOI: 10.3390/pharmaceutics15092253

[98] Ha SW, Viggeswarapu M, Habib MM, Beck GR Jr. Bioactive effects of silica nanoparticles on bone cells are size, surface, and composition dependent. Acta Biomaterialia. 2018;**82**:184-196.

Epub 20181014. DOI: 10.1016/j.actbio.2018.10.018

[99] Jugdaohsingh R, Calomme MR, Robinson K, Nielsen F, Anderson SH, D'Haese P, et al. Increased longitudinal growth in rats on a silicon-depleted diet. Bone. 2008;**43**:596-606. Epub 20080502. DOI: 10.1016/j.bone.2008.04.014

[100] Kostka K, Hosseini S, Epple M. In-vitro cell response to strontium/magnesium-doped calcium phosphate nanoparticles. Micro. 2023;**3**:156-171. DOI: 10.3390/micro3010012

[101] Omidian H, Chowdhury SD. Advancements and applications of injectable hydrogel composites in biomedical research and therapy. Gels. 2023;**9**:533. Epub 20230630. DOI: 10.3390/gels9070533

[102] Zhu Y, Wang Y, Jia Y, Xu J, Chai Y. Catalpol promotes the osteogenic differentiation of bone marrow mesenchymal stem cells via the Wnt/beta-catenin pathway. Stem Cell Research & Therapy. 2019;**10**:37. Epub 20190122. DOI: 10.1186/s13287-019-1143-y

[103] Poulose A, Parameswaranpillai J, George JJ, Gopi JA, Krishnasamy S, Dominic CDM, et al. Nanocellulose: A fundamental material for science and technology applications. Molecules. 2022;**27**:1-27. Epub 20221119. DOI: 10.3390/molecules27228032

[104] Hossain N, Mobarak MH, Hossain A, Khan F, Mim JJ, Chowdhury MA. Advances of plant and biomass extracted zirconium nanoparticles in dental implant application. Heliyon. 2023;**9**:e15973. Epub 20230506. DOI: 10.1016/j.heliyon.2023.e15973

[105] Chowdhury MA, Hossain N, Mostofa MG, Mia MR, Tushar M, Rana MM, et al. Green synthesis and characterization of zirconium nanoparticlefor dental implant applications. Heliyon. 2023;**9**:e12711. Epub 20221230. DOI: 10.1016/j.heliyon.2022.e12711

[106] Motornov M, Malynych SZ, Pippalla DS, Zdyrko B, Royter H, Roiter Y, et al. Field-directed self-assembly with locking nanoparticles. Nano Letters. 2012;**12**:3814-3820. Epub 20120625. DOI: 10.1021/nl301780x

[107] Shankar SS, Rai A, Ahmad A, Sastry M. Rapid synthesis of Au, Ag, and bimetallic Au core-Ag shell nanoparticles using neem (Azadirachta indica) leaf broth. Journal of Colloid and Interface Science. 2004;**275**:496-502. DOI: 10.1016/j.jcis.2004.03.003

[108] Ankamwar B, Damle C, Ahmad A, Sastry M. Biosynthesis of gold and silver nanoparticles using Emblica Officinalis fruit extract, their phase transfer and transmetallation in an organic solution. Journal of Nanoscience and Nanotechnology. 2005;**5**:1665-1671. DOI: 10.1166/jnn.2005.184

[109] Li W, Qu F, Chen Y, Sun Y, Zhang J, Xie G, et al. Antimicrobial activity of sliver nanoparticles synthesized by the leaf extract of Cinnamomum camphora. Biochemical Engineering Journal. 2021;**172**:108050. DOI: 10.1016/j.bej.2021.108050

[110] Nava OJ, Luque PA, Gómez-Gutiérrez CM, Vilchis-Nestor AR, Castro-Beltrán A, Mota-González ML, et al. Influence of Camellia sinensis extract on zinc oxide nanoparticle green synthesis. Journal of Molecular Structure. 2017;**1134**:121-125. DOI: 10.1016/j.molstruc.2016.12.069

[111] Sirelkhatim A, Mahmud S, Seeni A, Kaus NHM, Ann LC, Bakhori SKM, et al.

Review on zinc oxide nanoparticles: Antibacterial activity and toxicity mechanism. Nano-micro Letters. 2015;**7**:219-242. Epub 20150419. DOI: 10.1007/s40820-015-0040-x

[112] Dayanandan AP, Cho WJ, Kang H, Bello AB, Kim BJ, Arai Y, et al. Emerging nano-scale delivery systems for the treatment of osteoporosis. Biomaterials Research. 2023;**27**:68. Epub 20230713. DOI: 10.1186/s40824-023-00413-7

[113] Cheng H, Chawla A, Yang Y, Li Y, Zhang J, Jang HL, et al. Development of nanomaterials for bone-targeted drug delivery. Drug Discovery Today. 2017;**22**:1336-1350. Epub 20170506. DOI: 10.1016/j.drudis.2017.04.021

[114] Liang W, Ding P, Li G, Lu E, Zhao Z. Hydroxyapatite nanoparticles facilitate osteoblast differentiation and bone formation within sagittal suture during expansion in rats. Drug Design, Development and Therapy. 2021;**15**:905-917. Epub 20210301. DOI: 10.2147/DDDT.S299641

[115] Alegrete N, Sousa SR, Padrao T, Carvalho A, Lucas R, Canadas RF, et al. Vancomycin-loaded, nanohydroxyapatite-based scaffold for osteomyelitis treatment: In vivo rabbit toxicological tests and In vivo efficacy tests in a sheep model. Bioengineering (Basel). 2023;**10**:1-19. Epub 20230204. DOI: 10.3390/bioengineering10020206